Anti-D in Midwifery: I

CW01022099

For Mum and Dad, with love

Commissioning editor: Mary Seager
Desk editor: Deena Burgess
Production controller: Chris Jarvis
Editorial assistant: Caroline Savage
Cover designer: Helen Brockway

Anti-D in Midwifery: Panacea or Paradox?

SARA WICKHAM, MA, BA(HONS), RM

For where is the man [sic] that has incontestable
evidence of the truth of all that he holds, or of the
falsehood of all he condemns, or can say that he
has examined to the bottom all his own, or other
men's, opinions? The necessity of believing without
knowledge, nay often upon very slight grounds, in
this fleeting state of action and blindness we are in,
should make us more busy and careful to inform
ourselves than constrain others.

John Locke, c. 1689, cited in Magee (1988)

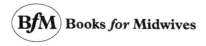 **Books *for* Midwives**

OXFORD AUCKLAND BOSTON JOHANNESBURG MELBOURNE NEW DELHI

Books for Midwives
An imprint of Butterworth-Heinemann
Linacre House, Jordan Hill, Oxford OX2 8DP
225 Wildwood Avenue, Woburn, MA 01801-2041
A division of Reed Educational and Professional Publishing Ltd

A member of the Reed Elsevier plc group

First published 2001
Transferred to digital printing 2004
© Sara Wickham 2001

All rights reserved. No part of this publication may be reproduced in
any material form (including photocopying or storing in any medium by
electronic means and whether or not transiently or incidentally to some
other use of this publication) without the written permission of the
copyright holder except in accordance with the provisions of the Copyright,
Designs and Patents Act 1988 or under the terms of a licence issued by the
Copyright Licensing Agency Ltd, 90 Tottenham Court Road, London,
England W1P 0LP. Applications for the copyright holder's written
permission to reproduce any part of this publication should be addressed
to the publishers

British Library Cataloguing in Publication Data
Wickham, Sara
    Anti-D in midwifery: panacea or paradox?
    1. Erythroblastosis fetalis – Prevention   2. Pregnancy –
    Complications   3. Blood products – Therapeutic use
    I. Title
    618.3′2′061

ISBN 0 7506 5232 2

Typeset by Avocet Typeset, Brill, Aylesbury, Bucks

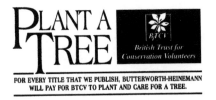

FOR EVERY TITLE THAT WE PUBLISH, BUTTERWORTH-HEINEMANN
WILL PAY FOR BTCV TO PLANT AND CARE FOR A TREE.

Contents

Acknowledgements

I owe thanks to a number of people who have supported me in this project:

To my parents, who have supported me in all manner of ways throughout the entire process of researching and writing; special thanks to my mum for proofreading the entire manuscript.

To Mark Horridge and Martin Pooley, whose expert help in the field of haematology and willingness to debate the issues herein proved invaluable.

To my midwife (and honorary midwife) colleagues who have shared their time, expertise and resources; Lorna Davies, Judy Edmunds, Anne Gridley, Valerie El Halta, Michel Odent, Mary Stewart, Jan Tritten and Naoli Vinaver.

To Huguette Comerasamy, Robbie Davis-Floyd and Jon Burke for providing academic support and advice during the original research upon which this book is based.

To the midwives and midwifery students who have heard me speak on these issues and who have, by asking the right questions, helped expand the boundaries of my own thinking.

To a small army of friends and colleagues who helped in all kinds of ways, from finding research papers and being willing to listen without sounding bored to taking me in for weekends at just the right time; Debbie and Richard Willett, Fiona MacIntosh and Ian Peters, Juan Carlos Frietman, Janice Marsh-Prelesnik, Janice Bass, Jenny Green, Jan Bliss, Margo Fyfe, Maggie Cook, Mike Taylor, Susie, Molly and Tish Poppy.

Finally, to the midwives and women, who gave so freely of their time and philosophies, who have retained a sense of power in their own bodies, and who care enough to challenge.

CHAPTER ONE

Introduction and background

For a number of years, midwives and other birth attendants have been embracing a philosophy of evidence-informed practice. Most of the medical interventions that have become a routine part of women's care during pregnancy and birth have been examined in the light of research findings and other evidence. Evaluation of the benefits, risks and effectiveness of a wide range of interventions, including artificial rupture of the membranes, episiotomy and electronic fetal monitoring, has taken place over the last two decades. One of the major outcomes of much of this research has been that, when held up to close scrutiny, most of the interventions introduced into normal childbirth through the process of medicalization have been discovered to be futile, and often potentially harmful, when used on a routine basis.

There remains one, however, that does not appear to have been challenged by midwife (or other) researchers to date; the routine administration of anti-D immunoglobulin (anti-D) to rhesus-negative mothers following the birth of a rhesus-positive baby. It is this topic that I have been researching for 3 years, and will be discussing in this book. (For those who are unfamiliar with anti-D, or exactly what this does, there is an outline of the issues towards the end of this chapter.)

My interest in this topic derived from practice as well as academic experience; as an independent midwife I worked with women who, having read the literature on medical interventions in childbirth, actively chose to avoid these where possible. For some women, this avoidance extended to postnatal anti-D. Prior to this experience I had read reviews of the research evidence in this area, which were unequivocal in their conclusion that anti-D was necessary for all women in this situation and might also be advisable as a routine intervention during pregnancy. I became acutely aware of the discrepancy between this evidence and the concept of normality during the birth process. As a midwife, this led me to question my practice and the information I gave women.

Working with these women highlighted the paradox that seemed to exist in this area. On the one hand, analysis of almost all of the research and other evidence concerned with birth confirms that this is a normal and physiological process, which works far better without routine intervention. However, it is difficult to reconcile this with the current knowledge base surrounding anti-D, which suggests that the administration of this product to rhesus-negative women who have given birth to a rhesus-positive baby is essential to prevent them producing their own anti-D, which may be potentially harmful to future babies. If birth works better for the vast majority of the time without intervention, then what makes anti-D the proverbial exception to the rule?

By raising this question I am not denying the life-saving nature of anti-D; as one of the medical world's success stories, anti-D may have saved the lives of hundreds or thousands of babies since its discovery and introduction. Few people would question the place of such a product in modern maternity care, or the importance of the work that has been carried out in this area. Yet it is precisely because few people were questioning the need for anti-D that it seemed important to research this area. In order to make progress, we must be able to ask those questions that are uncomfortable. In fact, I would suggest that these questions may be among the most important.

Anti-D: explaining and defining the issue

Before discussing the process of research undertaken here, a basic outline of the issues concerning rhesus grouping and an overview of the current 'received view' in the area follows. Our present understanding of this area sits quite firmly within the biochemical model of childbirth, and tends to assume that all rhesus-negative women will potentially have the problems described.

There are several methods of categorizing blood types, the most commonly known being the ABO system, in which humans may have blood types A, B, AB or O. As well as being one of these types, blood is classified according to whether the 'rhesus factor' is present or absent. It is important to note that the term 'rhesus' does not only apply to the rhesus D factor, which is the one discussed in this book, but also to the less common C and E forms. Strictly speaking, Rh D-negative (rather than the more general rhesus negative) is the most accurate term to use when discussing this issue. However, for the purpose of this book the terms rhesus, rhesus positive and rhesus negative are used for ease of reading, and the reader is asked to assume that these all apply to the D form of the rhesus factor.

About 85 per cent of Caucasians have blood that contains a protein known as the rhesus factor; they are termed rhesus-positive (Rh D-positive). The presence of the rhesus D factor is represented in medical shorthand by the capital letter 'D'. The remaining 15 per cent do not have this factor, and their blood is described as being rhesus-negative (Rh D-negative). The absence of the rhesus factor is denoted by a small 'd'. The only way to determine the presence or absence of this factor is by a blood test. The rates of rhesus-positive and rhesus-negative people vary with ethnicity (see Chapter 6 for further discussion of this point).

People who have the rhesus factor are never compromised by this. However, if a person who is rhesus negative comes into contact with the rhesus factor (for instance by receiving a blood transfusion containing this), there may be consequences. In simple terms, the blood will recognize the rhesus factor as foreign and produce antibodies which help remove it from the person's system. These antibodies remain in the body and enable the person to 'fight off' further rhesus factor in the future. This process can be compared with having a cold or infection; the body's immune system 'fights off' the foreign substance and produces antibodies which ensure that, if the body encounters the same substance again, it will be able to fight the infection effectively. The issue here is what happens when a rhesus-negative woman comes into contact with rhesus-positive blood from her baby.

In pregnancy, the mother's and baby's blood do not usually mix; their vessels are kept separate by means of the placenta, which allows the nutrients and oxygen to pass from the mother to the baby while at the same time allowing the carbon dioxide and waste substances to be removed. However, it is possible that, either during pregnancy or around the time of birth, a small amount of the baby's blood can leak into the mother's bloodstream. If the baby's blood is also rhesus negative, nothing will happen as a result of this, even if the ABO type is different. The rhesus factor is absent and no problems will ensue. However, if the baby is rhesus positive and some of the blood leaks into the rhesus-negative mother's bloodstream, the mother's blood will recognize it as foreign and may produce anti-D antibodies against it. This process is known as isoimmunization, and takes several days. Once isoimmunization has occurred, the mother may be described as 'sensitized'. Although this is a mechanism designed to protect the mother, it can have a detrimental effect on any future rhesus-positive babies she has.

This problem will not affect a woman's first baby unless isoimmunization has occurred previously (such as from a mismatched blood transfusion, or at the time of an abortion or miscarriage). However, if rhesus antibodies are produced, subsequent rhesus-positive babies may be affected because the antibodies are able to cross the membrane at the placenta (even though actual blood cannot) and may attack the rhesus proteins in the baby's blood. This can cause a range of problems, from mild jaundice to severe rhesus haemolytic disease, which in the worst cases can result in the death of the baby. Although a far greater proportion of babies suffering from rhesus disease survive nowadays as a result of advances in care, they may require blood transfusions, early delivery or intensive care.

'Anti-D' is also the name given to a manufactured substance that can be given to the mother when the risk of isoimmunization is thought to be significant, such as immediately after the birth of a rhesus-positive baby. It is derived from the blood of donors who have been isoimmunized as a result of receiving rhesus-positive blood either accidentally (e.g. during pregnancy or a blood transfusion) or, more usually, deliberately (with the sole purpose of making their blood available for the manufacture of this product). The antibodies in the artificial anti-D will 'fight off' any rhesus-positive cells from the baby and prevent the woman from producing her own anti-D.

The history of anti-D

Many of the issues surrounding the administration of anti-D may be more clearly viewed in an historical context, and the following outlines the development of ideas and research in this area.

The condition of haemolytic disease of the newborn was discussed by Plato and has been occasionally documented since the seventeenth century, although it was not until 1938 that scientists suggested this might be caused by an immune reaction in the mother to paternal factors carried by the developing baby (Howard et al., 1997a).

Once scientists had identified the rhesus factor as being a protein that is present in some people's blood but not in others, Levine et al. (1941) were able to describe the process of isoimmunization. As explained above, this occurs where maternal antibodies are formed in response to antigen from the fetus. Although paediatric care had reached the stage where many of the babies suffering from the effects of this condition could be helped, the general feeling was that there was still a need to prevent maternal sensitization (Howard et al., 1997a) and thus stop the problem before it occurred.

Initially, work was carried out to study the nature of the protection that seemed to be offered to women when their blood group differed from that of the baby they were carrying. Research into this situation of ABO incompatibility between mother and baby led to the proposition by Clarke et al. (1963) that the administration of intramuscular anti-D immunoglobulin cleared fetal red cells from the maternal circulation and prevented rhesus isoimmunization in women. Specific details of the clinical trials set up to test this proposition are discussed in Chapter 2.

As a result of these trials, which were considered to have proved the theory that artificial anti-D was effective in preventing isoimmunization, anti-D was produced and the recommendation made that this should be administered to all rhesus-negative women who had given birth to a rhesus-positive baby (or one where the rhesus group was undetermined). This policy has remained largely unchanged to the present day, with more recent research focusing on the specific dose required and the issue of antenatal administration.

Current use of anti-D

The current recommendations for the use of anti-D suggest that it should be routinely offered to a rhesus-negative mother within 72 hours of the birth of a rhesus-positive baby. A Kleihauer test (see Chapter 2) is usually performed concurrently to establish whether a woman needs more than the standard dose of anti-D. Anti-D should also be offered to women who experience a 'sensitizing event' in pregnancy; this may be an intervention (such as amniocentesis) or an accidental event (such as abdominal trauma or vaginal bleeding) which carries a risk of fetomaternal transfusion. In some areas, women will be offered anti-D routinely during pregnancy as well as after sensitizing events and the birth of their baby. This is not yet the case in the whole of the UK, although it is in some other countries, such as the USA.

So what is the woman's experience of these events? All women will be offered a blood test in early pregnancy in order to determine their blood group and rhesus status. (It should be noted that, in practice, most women do not realize that this test and its consequences are optional, and will generally go along with what they are told they need by professionals.) The woman may or may not be advised of the results of this test. Ideally, if a woman is found to be rhesus negative she should be told about this and given information about the pros and cons of anti-D so that she can make her own decision well ahead of time. She should also be informed about potentially sensitizing events so that she can request anti-D if she feels she needs it, rather than relying totally on this being picked up by clinicians. It is probably fair to say that the women who receive this kind of information are in the minority.

When the woman's baby is born, her blood will again be tested, as will that of her baby. If the baby is rhesus negative, no action will be taken. If the baby is rhesus positive, the results of the test will be returned to the woman's midwife, along with a vial containing the appropriate dose of anti-D. The midwife will approach the woman with the news that she needs anti-D, and this is usually administered (by intramuscular injection) without the woman receiving further information about the product or her individual need for it.

Few women question their need for anti-D, perhaps because, for myriad reasons, they do not realize that they have a choice about whether or not they receive it. However, a small but significant proportion of women have begun to question their own need for anti-D and to search for evidence regarding whether this is truly essential for them. While it might seem from the issues discussed above that anti-D is a wholly positive discovery offering only benefit to women and babies, several issues are causing concern to these women and to midwives.

The first and perhaps most important question concerns possible side effects of the product. The known and documented side effects listed by the manufacturers and pharmaceutical guidelines include local inflammation, malaise, chills, fever and, rarely, anaphylaxis. Some women have reported suffering an intensely irritating rash covering all or a large part of their body following administration of anti-D. Further concerns include those of immune system compromise and the issue of some pharmaceutical companies using a mercury-based preservative, which some women are actively choosing to avoid because of potential toxicity.

The second issue is that of blood-borne infections. Anti-D is a blood product, and as such has the potential to carry such infections. The risks of anti-D in this area are compounded by the fact that the blood used to make the product is pooled, so blood from one infected donor may end up in several hundred doses of the product. Several years ago, over 3000 women in Ireland contracted hepatitis C from infected anti-D (Meisel et al., 1995), and HIV has also been transmitted through anti-D (Dumasia et al., 1989). While both of these viruses are now screened for and would be rendered harmless by the purification processes involved, the most pressing concern relates to the presence of as yet unknown viruses, which may not be killed by current treatments. We can clearly only screen for and treat anti-D for those viruses that we know about and have the effective means to treat.

While an understanding of the reported side effects of anti-D is useful to women who are seeking to make an informed choice, there remains anxiety about the unknown risks of anti-D. No long-term research has been carried out into the effects of anti-D on women, babies in utero (when antenatal administration is offered) or subsequent babies. Although I have observed anecdotal discussion between midwives as to the potential implications of mass administration both for individual women and the population as a whole, this issue has not been adequately explored or researched.

Finally, the philosophical question is emerging as an issue for women. As more women learn that their bodies were designed to give birth, and gain a spirit of trust rather than the fear that has come to dominate birth in Western society, they and their midwives begin to question the need for any routine intervention in a natural process. Some women find it difficult to envisage why anti-D is necessary in a process that has been designed or created to work without intervention the vast majority of the time.

Raising questions and finding answers

It was these concerns and the paradox between the concept of physiological birth and the need for anti-D that led me to carry out a series of research projects. Initially I undertook a literature search to determine whether postnatal anti-D really was proven necessary for all rhesus-negative women who had given birth to a rhesus-positive baby. This highlighted the very real problem with the medical evidence; that, while anti-D was shown to be effective on a population basis, the very research which proved this also clearly showed that it was not necessary for most women in this situation. Following up the other issues raised by this search enabled me to uncover some of the risks of anti-D, the controversy surrounding routine antenatal administration of this and, perhaps more importantly, the lack of evidence regarding short- or long-term safety for women and babies.

Later I undertook primary research into the midwifery body of knowledge in this area, and began to explore with midwives what their experiences, feelings, thoughts and knowledge were in this area. I discovered that rather than there being only one viewpoint in this area (the medical stance already highlighted), there was also a body of knowledge that could be seen as fitting into the midwifery model and paradigm.

My research has continued as I have talked to women, midwives and other professionals around the world about the issue, and this book is the result of that process. I would like to emphasize that it is by no means intended as a 'final answer'; the research into this area is only just beginning, and there are many issues that still need exploration. Nor will the information presented necessarily make decisions any easier for women to make; there are no fail-safe answers. There is, however, a need for discussion, exploration and reflection on the issues.

The first section of this book comprises analysis of the existing research published in this area. Chapter 2 summarizes the evidence offered by clinical trials, and considers questions relating to the routine postnatal administration of anti-D. Chapter 3 considers subsequent research relating to wider issues in the area, including those of dosage, virus transmission and the effectiveness of the current programme. The issue of antenatal anti-D, evidence for and against this and the current professional and political debate in this area is discussed in Chapter 4.

Chapter 5 outlines the process of the research I undertook in order to try to discover whether previously unrecorded midwifery knowledge existed in this area, while Chapters 6–10 discuss the results of this study. Chapter 6 considers the philosophical differences between the midwives and existing views in this area. Clinical and immunological factors that midwives feel might be important in determining whether a particular woman needs anti-D are discussed in Chapter 7, while Chapter 8 considers one of these factors, the physiology of the placenta and third stage of labour, in depth. Chapter 9 comprises a number of positive intercessions suggested by midwives to offer protection against fetomaternal haemorrhage, and Chapter 10 considers the debate concerning informed choice, and the information that women need in this area.

The final chapters focus around the continuation of the debate surrounding anti-D. The differences between the midwifery and medical paradigms highlighted by work in this area are discussed in Chapter 11, while Chapter 12 concludes the book by considering how we can best use the knowledge gained through this process and move midwifery knowledge forward on a wider and more general basis.

A glossary is included at the back of this book for those who may not be familiar with all of the terms used, along with a bibliography containing details of the references cited within the text.

CHAPTER TWO

Initial research

The first stage of evaluation of the knowledge base in a given area is to analyse as much of the existing research in that area as possible. In order to try to throw some light on the paradox between women's capacity for physiological birth and their need for anti-D, this chapter outlines the trials conducted to test the proposition that anti-D prevents isoimmunization and other research that impacts on and adds to our knowledge concerning the need for postnatal anti-D as a routine intervention.

Research methodology

As discussed in Chapter 1, the decision to administer anti-D to all rhesus-negative women who gave birth to a rhesus-positive baby was made in the light of the evidence gained from the clinical trials of this product. A literature search revealed that nine major clinical trials were carried out around the world between 1967 and 1971 to test the effectiveness of anti-D.

In order to evaluate these research trials, a research protocol was developed. This protocol (shown in Table 2.1) contained five criteria which, when applied to the clinical trials, would enable an assessment to be made of the methodological strength of each trial. A trial that meets most (or all) of the criteria would be likely to be more accurate (less potentially biased) than a trial that did not meet any of the criteria. The criteria set in this case were: including appropriate women as subjects; randomization of women; double-blinding of the intervention; appropriately large numbers of women;

and independent funding rather than pharmaceutical company sponsorship. Table 2.2 shows the specific details of the trials in relation to each of these criteria.

Table 2.1 Research protocol

Aspect of methodology	Notes
Appropriate subjects	All rhesus-negative women who had given birth to rhesus-positive babies. This would give information on the entire population figures before any breakdown occurred due to other factors
Appropriate number of subjects	At least 100 women in each of the study and control groups. This number may be too small when considering adverse outcomes; however, it acknowledges that the rate of rhesus immunization may be detectable even with quite small numbers
Effective randomization	Women should be assigned to study or control groups purely on the basis of chance. Neither the researcher nor the woman should elect which group is entered. The method of randomization should be made explicit and adhered to during the study
Double blinding of intervention	Neither the women nor the researcher should know to which group they have been assigned. This implies that a placebo should be used for women in the control group
Sources of funding	Although it was not intended that this would imply exclusion of studies, the sponsor of the research would be noted as a possible source of bias

Consideration of these criteria was an important part of the process, as the way in which these trials were carried out raises a number of issues. Generally, in order for a trial to be considered unbiased, women in such a study need to be randomly allocated to one of the

Table 2.2 Application of research protocol to clinical trials of anti-D

Study and location	Appropriate subjects	Appropriate number of subjects	Effective randomization	Double blinding	Sponsor
Ascari et al. (1968), International	yes	yes i = 1081 c = 675	?	no	Ortho
Bishop and Krieger (1969), Australia	?	yes i = 121 c = 131	?	no	Ortho
Chown et al. (1969), W. Canada	?	yes i = 1216 c = 500	?	no	?
Clarke et al. (1971), UK/USA	no (used 'high risk' women)	no i = 86 c = 65	?	no	?
Dudok de Wit et al. (1968), Holland	yes	yes i = 333 c = 329	quasi-random	no	?
Robertson and Holmes (1969), Edinburgh	? 'at risk' women	yes i = 100 c = 112	quasi-random (also changed during study)	no	?
Stenchever et al. (1970), USA	yes	no i = 26 c = 28	yes	yes	?
White et al. (1970), USA	yes	yes i = 160 c = 153	yes	yes	?
Woodrow et al. (1971), Liverpool	no 'low risk' women	yes i = 353 c = 362	yes	no	?

i, intervention group; c, control group; ?, study did not give enough information to answer question; Ortho, Ortho Pharmaceuticals (a company that produces and sells anti-D).

groups; in this case, those who received anti-D or those who didn't. Well-conducted clinical trials also need to utilize double-blinding, where neither the woman nor the researchers know who is in which group. Double-blinding is often achieved by the use of a placebo pill or injection that is given to women in the control group; this must resemble the product being tested, but is inert. When randomization and double-blinding are used, the researchers (and those reading the research) can be confident that bias did not enter the trial in this way. Otherwise, the women's or clinician's preconceptions of the product being tested may subconsciously influence the data in some way.

Neither of these techniques was used in the majority of the clinical trials for anti-D. In fact, two of the later groups of researchers (Stenchever *et al.*, 1970; White *et al.*, 1970) designed studies in response to what the authors felt were the methodological short-comings of initial work in this area, namely that randomization and double-blinding had not been utilized. One of these trials (Stenchever *et al.*, 1970) was stopped after only 54 women had been entered because anti-D was made available for all women on the basis of previous research. In some ways this was unfortunate, because the preliminary results of this trial appeared to show that anti-D was less effective than the results of the other trials had suggested. The other trial (White *et al.*, 1970) also showed interesting results; 313 women took part and the isoimmunization rate in the control group was the lowest of all of the nine clinical trials. It is impossible to know whether these results were a more accurate representation of the effectiveness of anti-D because randomization and double-blinding was used, or whether (particularly in the case of the Stenchever *et al.* trial) they were less accurate because not enough women had been entered in the trials to make a fair assessment of the effectiveness of anti-D.

It seems that stopping the research or changing the subject of the trial was not uncommon in this field; the Medical Research Council set up a working party in 1966 to evaluate the effectiveness of anti-D and a clinical trial was started. However, as the researchers watched the results of other trials emerge, they realized that these were showing anti-D to be effective, and changed the entire nature of their own trial before it was completed. Where initially they had not given women in the control group any anti-D, they began to give these women a 'relatively small but potentially effective dose of anti-

D' (Mollison *et al.*, 1974). The numbers of women in the groups were small and the results of this trial never published, as a larger study then took place (this study is discussed further in Chapter 3).

These examples of groups of researchers changing or ceasing their studies before completion raise some interesting issues. While the ideal of scientific research is to ensure that findings are replicable – that is, the same results would be achieved from similar studies – the decisions to stop these studies meant that further data was lost to the field. Ultimately, the studies in question had so few participants that the data was difficult to quantify and is not nearly as valuable as if they had continued with a larger number of participants. While they were stopped essentially for altruistic reasons, in that it was perhaps felt unethical not to give anti-D to the women in the control groups when this had been shown to be effective, the net result is that we are left with less than optimal data in the field as a whole.

The second question that this action suggests is this: to what degree were the trials conducted independently? It may be more valuable to run several independent research projects; if the results of these agree with each other, we can be more certain that the data are reliable and valid. However, more than one group of researchers on the anti-D project are acknowledging that they changed their own research on the basis of the findings of others. What if the findings of the first study were inaccurate in some way? Would the other groups be more likely to look for the same findings? Would it be more appropriate to consider the research as one or more world-wide collaborative research projects rather than a greater number of independent trials?

The research protocol that I developed to evaluate the original trials (Table 2.1) was intended to highlight potential bias. After applying this protocol, I discovered that several of the studies may have been subject to some form of bias. This does not imply that the results are invalid, but that they may need to be treated with caution. For instance, at least three of the nine trials were funded by the pharmaceutical company that produced anti-D; although this is common for drug trials, it does beg the question of whether there may have been inappropriate influence on the research.

If, as suggested above, some degree of collaboration occurred between those conducting the trials, then to what degree would the fact that some of the trials were being funded by pharmaceutical companies affect or influence the results? Could some of the results of these studies be less independent than we might think? In several cases, the paper simply does not give enough information to make an objective assessment of methodological quality, although it should be acknowledged that these studies were undertaken when the knowledge base concerning research methods was not as broad as it is today.

Determining the effectiveness of anti-D

The results of the trials showed that, on a population basis, anti-D was effective in preventing rhesus isoimmunization. The vast majority of women in the groups that received anti-D did not become isoimmunized or go on to develop antibodies to the rhesus antigen. The results clearly showed anti-D to be effective: 0.2 per cent (6/2973) of women in the groups receiving anti-D were sensitized at 6 months postpartum, compared to 7.5 per cent (186/2488) of women in control groups.

The trials that looked at the rate of sensitization – apparently in some of the same women – in a subsequent pregnancy also showed that women receiving anti-D were much less likely to be sensitized. However, only five of the original trials published data in this category, and none of these included more than 260 women in total; in fact, one (White et al., 1970) included only 21 women. Even a trial with 130 women in each group would be considered by some researchers to be too small to provide reliable results.

The suggestion that the data pertaining to isoimmunization in subsequent pregnancy may not be accurate seems to be borne out by closer analysis of the results. In both the intervention and control groups in the largest of these trials (Woodrow et al., 1971), a higher proportion of women were sensitized than would have been expected from previous data: 2.34 per cent (3/128) of women in the intervention group, and 10.24 per cent (13/137) of women in the control group. These results suggest that anti-D is less effective in the long term than first thought. However, more recent data suggesting that postnatal anti-D administration is effective in 99 per cent of the population (Tovey, 1992) refute this, which would tend to support the theory that the trials that looked at the rate of isoimmunization in a subsequent pregnancy were not methodologically sound enough to be considered as valid evidence. It then follows that the proportion of women sensitized in the control groups may also not be accurate.

One of the implications of this concerns the idea of sensibilization, which describes the process where a woman may be exposed to the rhesus antigen but not develop antibodies to it. In other words, it has been suggested that some women may not show antibodies upon testing at 6 months postpartum, but that these may still develop in a subsequent pregnancy where the baby is rhesus positive. This process has been described by a number of researchers (Woodrow et al., 1971; Bowman and Pollock, 1978), and forms part of the current medical opinion in this area. Yet if the data on which this supposition is based may be inaccurate, then surely this should be tested again in order to determine whether sensibilization is a real risk to rhesus-negative women and, if so, how often this really occurs.

In considering the effectiveness of anti-D, the groups of researchers did not look at other variables in relation to the likelihood of isoimmunization. It may be that the effectiveness (or indeed the need for) this product is mitigated by other factors, including pre-existing clinical conditions or the use of other drugs around the time of birth. However, the clinical trials do not give enough information to enable further hypotheses to be formulated. Furthermore, in his review of the issues for the *Effective Care in Pregnancy and Childbirth* project, Bennebrock Gravenhorst (1989) concluded that factors other than use of anti-D have been involved in the decline of rhesus disease. The most relevant of these is almost certainly the trend towards smaller families; before anti-D, rhesus disease often did not manifest until the third or fourth child (Howard et al., 1997b). Improved maternal and neonatal care is also considered to have impacted on this situation.

Determining the necessity for anti-D

It is clear from the nature of this research that it did not attempt to determine whether anti-D is necessary for individual women. The trials studied the effectiveness of anti-D in preventing rhesus isoimmunization in populations of rhesus-negative women. While the strength of randomized controlled trials lies in seeing the 'bigger picture' of causal relationships, their weakness in this context is that it is difficult to extrapolate information about the need for anti-D for individual woman.

The data from the trials do suggest that anti-D is not necessary for all women; between 1.96 per cent (3/153; White *et al.*, 1970) and 13.39 per cent (15/112; Robertson and Holmes, 1969) of women in the control groups were isoimmunized at 6 months. Overall, the average rate of isoimmunization of women in control groups was 7.5 per cent (186/2488), which implies that around 90 per cent of women may not need anti-D. No research has yet considered why, on average, only 10 per cent of women need anti-D while 90 per cent of rhesus-negative women who give birth to a rhesus-positive baby remain unaffected. It is impossible to predict from the clinical trials whether this is a detectable difference, whether protection is likely to be conferred by some pre-existing condition or whether it could be due to differences in transplacental haemorrhage or anti-body production following exposure to the rhesus antigen.

Additional anti-D

While the original clinical trials primarily considered the effectiveness of anti-D given following the birth of a rhesus-positive baby, it soon became clear that there were other situations where the administration of anti-D may be appropriate. The recommendations issued in 1969 on the basis of the evidence from the clinical trials were updated by the Standing Medical Advisory Committee in 1976; these now included the suggestion that a dose of anti-D should be given to all rhesus-negative women following miscarriage or abortion. In 1981, yet another recommendation was added; that anti-D should be offered to women who experienced 'potentially sensitizing events' in pregnancy (Standing Medical Advisory Committee, 1981). These events included accidental occurrences, such as abdominal trauma or vaginal bleeding, and medical interventions, including amniocentesis and external cephalic version.

The guidelines were then reviewed, in 1991, by the Immunoglobulin Working Party of the UK Blood Transfusion Service; this time, the review included guidance for clinicians concerning the administration of anti-D to rhesus-negative women who had accidentally been given rhesus-positive blood via transfusion. These guidelines, which essentially remained the same as those published when the programme started, were not reviewed again for several years, until a working group gathered in 1996 to reassess the 1991 regulations (Robson *et al.*, 1998). This group 'comprised obstetricians and haematologists with a special interest in rhesus disease' (Robson *et al.*, 1998). The main recommendations of the group concerned the administration of anti-D following sensitizing events in pregnancy, and the routine administration of anti-D in the antenatal period. This was quickly followed by the consensus conference on anti-D prophylaxis, held in Edinburgh in April 1997, to assess the evidence for routine antenatal anti-D prophylaxis; this conference is discussed in Chapter 4.

Transplacental haemorrhage

It seems unlikely from the research evidence that transplacental haemorrhage is inevitable at any stage of pregnancy or birth, although this is currently impossible to prove conclusively because of the nature of the testing involved. In order to determine whether fetal cells have crossed into the maternal circulation, haematologists perform a Kleihauer test. This test stains fetal blood cells a darker colour than maternal blood cells. Having added the dye, the operator smears a small sample of the woman's blood onto a slide and examines it under a microscope, and then looks at several 'fields' (or different parts of the slide) and counts the number of visible darker fetal cells. This number is then used to estimate the total amount of fetal cells that have entered the woman's bloodstream.

There are three main problems with the Kleihauer test. First, not all of the fetal cells pick up the dye, so the estimate may not be accurate; this may also lead to variation between scientists, with higher estimates being made by some to compensate for the problem. Secondly, the test relies on the assumption that a random sample of a few millilitres of a woman's blood is representative of the much larger volume that circulates her body. Finally, the test is subject to human error, both in the estimation of the number of cells and the procedure used to carry the test out. Therefore, the Kleihauer test is at best a good estimate of the volume of fetal cells that have entered the woman's circulation.

Despite these issues, researchers generally agree that transplacental haemorrhage occurs in around 15 per cent of cases where a rhesus-negative woman carries a rhesus-positive baby (Zipursky and Israels, 1967; Woodrow *et al.*, 1971; Lachman *et al.*, 1977). In Zipursky and

Israels' (1967) study, 82.4 per cent of the women (980/1190) showed no fetal cells on Kleihauer testing. Unfortunately, the researchers did not separate this group from those women with a low but definitely positive Kleihauer when analysing results; we cannot then tell from their research what proportion of women (if any) with a negative Kleihauer went on to form antibodies. Their study did, however, show a clear link between the size of transplacental haemorrhage and the likelihood of isoimmunization, as did subsequent research by Woodrow et al. (1971).

It is not known whether the likelihood of transplacental haemorrhage can be correlated to maternal or birth-related factors, mainly because very little research has been carried out in this area. However, one study of its incidence during curettage following abortion found that trauma to the uterus increased its likelihood (Katz, 1969), and the same result might conceivably occur from intervention during birth. One small study (du Bois et al., 1991) showed that fetomaternal haemorrhage was more likely to occur in instrumental delivery and Caesarean section than in spontaneous birth; the rates of 'fetomaternal haemorrhage of clinical relevance' were 7.5 per cent for spontaneous delivery, 11.1 per cent for vacuum extraction and 17.7 per cent for Caesarean section. There were no differences between the rates of larger fetomaternal haemorrhage in different types of birth. Unfortunately, the number of women in this study was relatively small (391), and it may be inaccurate to consider the type of birth alone when other factors such as the use of oxytocic drugs may influence the likelihood of transplacental haemorrhage.

Antibody formation

There has been little research since the 1960s concerning the process by which isoimmunization occurs; the majority of work was carried out before anti-D was first manufactured. The assumption has been made that all rhesus-negative women have the potential to form rhesus antibodies. The initial work which identified that some protection was offered to the rhesus-negative women through ABO incompatibility was stopped after anti-D became available, as the potential of this research appeared 'unpromising' to the researchers (Ascari et al., 1969).

It has been assumed that transplacental haemorrhage automatically leads to antibody formation, although it has been shown that some women are more likely to produce antibodies following transplacental haemorrhage than others (Woodrow and Donahoe, 1968). The risk of antibody formation again rises with the volume of transplacental haemorrhage, as detected by Kleihauer testing.

Generally, the studies that claim to show that anti-D is effective often also provide evidence to support the theory that not all women need anti-D. In the study by Woodrow and Donahoe (1968), only 3.6 per cent (13/359) of women who had a negative Kleihauer had developed antibodies 6 months after the birth of their baby. These researchers surmised from the data collected at that time that, if anti-D had not developed within 6 months after delivery, it was unlikely to do so later. While their later study (Woodrow et al., 1971) included discussion of the risk of sensibilization, the existence of this phenomenon does not seem to be supported by the results of effective research.

Risks of routine anti-D administration

No research has been carried out into the long-term implications or potential risks of routine anti-D administration for either women or subsequent babies, despite the fact that this product has been administered to women for nearly 30 years. The original trials mentioned above only collected data on 3476 women who received anti-D, which is not a large number when trying to determine side effects – particularly those that are rare – and few of the studies specifically mention their findings in this area. While other studies have collected data on 10 000 women receiving anti-D (Crowther and Middleton, 1997), there has been no systematic effort to collect long-term data on the health of these women or their subsequent babies.

There is also little accessible evidence concerning reported adverse effects of this drug. Side effects listed in the product packaging include fever, chills, malaise, local inflammation, short-term discomfort at the injection site, and anaphylaxis (Bioproducts Laboratory, 1996). There is controversy about the potential risks of anti-D in certain areas, and a number of midwives have raised concerns about both the potential risks of anti-D and the information that women receive about these risks (Harmon, 1987; Gaskin, 1989; Wickham, 1999a).

As noted, concerns have been raised in relation to the transmission of the HIV (Dumasia, 1989) and hepatitis C (Meisel *et al.*, 1995) viruses in anti-D, although both of these viruses are now screened for. New variant Creutzfeldt Jakob disease (nvCJD) has become more of a concern in the UK in recent years, and this has led to the Department of Health's decision to stop using British blood supplies for plasma-derived products such as anti-D, instead buying blood and blood products from other countries. Interestingly, one of the countries from which the UK now purchases blood is the USA, where blood donors are paid for their efforts – a fact that has led critics to suggest that this 'market force' may lead to a lower quality of donated blood than that from unpaid voluntary donors.

Whatever the source of donated blood, the problem remains that the absolute risk of transmission of viral or other infectious material in blood products is unquantifiable because of the possibility of as yet undiscovered pathogens (Crowther and Middleton, 1997). It is only possible to screen blood for those viruses or pathogens of which we are aware, and can identify and destroy or render incapable of effect on humans.

Another concern is that anti-D may have negative effects on the reproductive health of subsequent babies, particularly girls, whose blood composition may be affected by the effects of the product on their mothers' immune system, DNA or blood composition. Although we currently have no concrete evidence of problems in this area, midwives have pointed out that only now are we seeing the first generation of women whose mothers were given anti-D giving birth, and it may therefore take time to identify any such problems. There is general agreement that further work needs to be undertaken to determine the risks and adverse effects of anti-D in women and subsequent babies (Crowther and Middleton, 1997; Bennebrock Gravenhorst, 1989).

Summarizing the issues

While Chapter 3 explores some of these issues in more depth, it can be seen from even a brief analysis of the initial data that the issues may not be as clear cut as we have come to believe. While anti-D was shown to be effective on a population basis, the clinical trials also show that it is potentially not necessary for all rhesus-negative women who have given birth to a rhesus-positive baby; less than 10 per cent of these women will need anti-D to prevent rhesus isoimmunization. We have little evidence that might help predict which women need anti-D; the product was given to all women on the strength of the trials, and no further research has been carried out to determine individual variations.

It has also been shown that transplacental haemorrhage is not inevitable during birth, and has been shown to occur in around 15 per cent of women. The risk of transplacental haemorrhage is increased with uterine trauma, and possibly other factors. Not all women who show evidence of transplacental haemorrhage will go on to develop antibodies. The risk of antibody development increases with the volume of fetomaternal transfusion, although it is not known whether there are factors which mitigate this risk. It may be important to note that much of the research discussed in this chapter was carried out on a population of women who were undergoing active management of their labour and birth, including the third stage. We do not know if this changed the rate of any of these factors from the 'baseline' level that would be seen in a population of women having 'natural' births. In other words, while less than 10 per cent of women experiencing medically managed birth will actually 'need' anti-D to prevent isoimmunization, it may be that even fewer women than this would need anti-D following physiological birth.

The historical context of this research is an important consideration. The decision was made to administer postnatal anti-D routinely to all rhesus-negative women with a rhesus-positive baby on the strength of the evidence produced by the clinical trials. At the time, the focus was on preventing rhesus disease in babies, and this was achieved. However, the results of the research clearly show that not all women need anti-D, although there was no attempt to determine whether this was predictable. The potential risks of anti-D, and strength of feeling from some women about this product, would suggest that further research into these areas is warranted.

The environment of maternity care has undergone myriad changes since the decision to administer anti-D on a routine basis was made. While the women who were giving birth in the early 1970s may not have felt they had much choice about their care, women in the twenty-first century are becoming more active in demanding their right to be making choices about their own and their babies' care.

There is a need to provide information for individual women, enabling them to make informed decisions about their own childbearing experience. It is clear that, in theory, not all rhesus-negative women who have given birth to a rhesus-positive baby will need postnatal anti-D, although in practice we currently have little information to offer women which will enable them to determine their own course of action.

CHAPTER THREE

Subsequent research

The main clinical trials of anti-D were completed by 1971, after which postnatal anti-D was administered routinely to rhesus-negative women who gave birth to a rhesus-positive baby in most areas of the Western world. Initially, anti-D was made available only to women having their first baby or to those who did not have any living children. Once supplies were sufficient, it was then offered to all women postnatally, according to national and local protocol.

There were – and remain – geographical differences between the protocols used in relation to routine postnatal anti-D. For example, while practitioners in some areas of the UK always perform blood tests on newborn babies in order to give postnatal anti-D only to women who have given birth to a rhesus-positive baby, others do not perform a blood test on the baby (perhaps because of the cost of this, or the timing of anti-D administration) and give anti-D to all rhesus-negative women regardless of their baby's blood group. In the time since postnatal anti-D became a routine intervention, research and discussion has been undertaken in a number of areas relating to the administration of anti-D. The aim of this chapter is to analyse and reflect upon some of this research.

How much anti-D?

The first large project following on from the clinical trials in the UK was that undertaken by the Medical Research Council (1974), who set up a working party in 1966 to consider and implement the most appropriate subsequent research studies. As discussed in Chapter 2, this is the group that changed the nature of their own clinical trial of anti-D to one that considered optimum dosage instead. The medical world in general seemed to have made the decision that anti-D was effective, and this may have been the crucial point at which the decisions as to how to continue in the field were made. The researchers would have been well aware that somewhere around 90 per cent of rhesus-negative women who carried a rhesus-positive baby did not need anti-D, and the option could have been to consider whether to conduct further studies to try to determine which women did and did not need anti-D. This option was clearly passed over in favour of administering anti-D to all women considered 'at risk'; the question now became how much anti-D those women should receive.

The Working Party's initial dosage trial results were not published, as the researchers considered that they 'added nothing material to those obtained in the main trial' (Mollison *et al.*, 1974). However, a larger trial then followed, which considered four different doses of anti-D; 20 mg, 50 mg, 100 mg and 200 mg. There were about 200 women in each of the dosage groups, and this trial was randomized and double-blinded. The researchers acknowledge that the doses were not exact; there seem to be a number of points where error could have occurred, and they estimate that the doses actually given were around 20 per cent higher than those stated. This is justified in the report of the trial by stating that it is not quite possible to inject the entire contents of the phial. It may be a matter of individual opinion as to whether this really is a justifiable position, or whether the results of the trial should be considered less than reliable as a result. In any case, the results failed to prove any differences between the effectiveness of the different doses, although the authors suggested that the dose of 20 mg should be considered sub-optimal.

At the time, the dose of anti-D generally given to women was 100 mg; in the absence of conclusive results this was continued, and remains the dose given today. (The current dose offered to women in the United Kingdom for routine postnatal prophylaxis is 500 iu, which equates to 100 mg.) It is considered that this is enough to clear the 'average' transplacental haemorrhage of up to 4 ml of fetal blood, and a Kleihauer test can be performed after the birth (or other potentially sensitizing event) to establish whether feto-maternal bleeding over this level has occurred, in which case further anti-D can be offered to clear the remaining fetal antibodies from the maternal circulation.

Reviewers of this evidence consider that we still do not have enough sound evidence concerning the optimal dosage of anti-D (Crowther and Middleton, 1997). While the dose given in Ireland, France and Canada is similar to that given in the UK, the standard dose in the USA is 1500 iu (300 mg). Most European countries other than France give 1000–1500 iu, or 200–300 mg (Howard et al., 1997b). This is a large difference, with women in the USA and parts of Europe receiving three times the dose that women in other parts of the world receive. This also has implications in terms of cost, supply and the potential risk of side effects.

It should be noted that we also do not have accurate information regarding the time scale in which doses of anti-D must be given to be effective; initial studies in this area were conducted among prisoners (most famously in Sing Sing Prison), where logistical constraints meant that the dosage was given within 72 hours of the rhesus-negative subject being injected with rhesus-positive blood (Romm, 1999). Today clinicians endeavour to give anti-D within this 72-hour window (which was shown to be effective), but without knowing how long after a transfusion of rhesus-positive blood anti-D would still be effective. There are women for whom this information may be particularly useful.

Howard et al. (1997a) further considered the issue of dosage in relation to the European Committee for Proprietary Medicinal Products' suggestion in 1992 that the routine administration of a larger postnatal dose of 1000–1500 iu would eradicate the need for routine Kleihauer testing to determine whether a woman needed more than the standard dose of 500 iu. While this suggestion might have been tabled as a cost-cutting exercise, a simple raising of the standard dosage of anti-D may not offer satisfactory protection for all women. Howard et al. (1997a) noted that this amount of anti-D would only cover a fetomaternal bleed of up to 15 ml, and referred to the study by Mollison et al. (1974) which showed that 0.3 per cent of women experience a bleed greater than this amount. The fact that these women would be unprotected while a much greater proportion of women would be exposed to far more anti-D than they required seems to suggest that this change is not beneficial. Despite this, some Trusts in the UK have changed their policies to give 1200 iu as the standard postnatal dose, although it is unclear whether they are ultimately proposing to eradicate the Kleihauer test.

While research in this area seems to have dwindled of late, optimum dosage may be a very important consideration for women. Few people want to receive a higher dose of any drug product than they need, especially if this might increase their risk of experiencing any side effects. This is also an important factor in the antenatal anti-D debate. Why are we not seeing research studies that continue to explore this question? Perhaps more importantly, why are we always so keen to find a dose that is optimal for the 'population', rather than finding a way to work out the specific volume of anti-D required by an individual?

Viral transmission

During the 1970s the anti-D project faced other problems, not least of which was the issue of virus transmission to women receiving anti-D. During 1978 and 1979, a single-source outbreak of hepatitis C occurred in 2533 Irish women who had received contaminated anti-D (Meisel *et al.*, 1995). This episode was followed by a handful of studies that followed up groups of women to assess whether hepatitis C and other viruses were being contracted from batches of the product (see discussions in *The Lancet*, 6 May and 13 May, 1995). Unfortunately, there is no central source of data on virus transmission, and it is impossible to determine the rate of viral transmission from anti-D because of the difficulty in tracing these data. Women are reassured by various sources that their risk of receiving virally-contaminated anti-D is low, but, although this may well be the case, the same women are not offered specific data so they can judge the risk for themselves, and decide whether it is one they are willing to take.

In 1994 a national screening programme was set up in Ireland in response to another cluster of hepatitis C cases, and Reilley and Lawlor (1999) reported the identification of a number of 'suspect batches' of anti-D. Clearly the 1978 outbreak was not an isolated episode, even for one country. The problem of virus transmission is not unique to anti-D; the Irish Blood Transfusion Board conducted a tribunal of enquiry into the cases, and found 'many other transmission episodes of hepatitis C virus by immunoglobulin preparations' (Yap, 1997). Anti-D is, however, the only immunoglobulin preparation routinely administered to healthy women of childbearing age.

Other forms of hepatitis have also been transmitted via anti-D; in the former East Germany there were cases of hepatitis B and non-A, non-B hepatitis contracted through contaminated anti-D (Kircheber *et al.*, 1994). This group of researchers, along with a number of others, sought to assess the extent of the problem by testing the blood of a group of randomly chosen women who had received anti-D since its introduction. They compared the presence of viruses in this group with those found in a group of rhesus-positive women, concluding that the fact that they found no statistically significant differences between the groups confirmed the viral safety of the products. However, this may be considered less convincing upon finding that the conclusion was made on the basis of blood tests on just 520 rhesus-negative women. Thus far, nobody has suggested that virus-contaminated anti-D is the norm; merely that batches of contaminated anti-D have been identified and that there is an occasional or potential risk of infection. With thousands of women receiving anti-D every year in any given country, the real surprise would be if a random sample of 520 women showed an incidence of viral transmission from any blood product. We need much better ways of measuring the incidence of viral transmission through anti-D or other products, and of storing these data in a way that is easily accessible to women and their caregivers. In this way, women could be given more accurate information regarding the risks of anti-D or similar products, and those responsible for monitoring such outbreaks would be able to identify contaminated product more quickly and remove it from use.

The HIV antibody has also been transmitted through anti-D in some countries (Dumasia *et al.*, 1989; Malviya *et al.*, 1989). Since it became understood that the HIV virus can be transmitted in plasma, routine screening of blood products has been undertaken in most countries. In the case of the UK, this was implemented in 1985 (Hoffbrand *et al.*, 1999). However, other countries were not so fast to react to developments in this area. Dumasia *et al.* (1989) confirmed that 'batches produced {in India} in late 1988 would have been administered to several Rh(D) negative women before the product was banned'. In fact, four contaminated batches were found to be HIV-antibody positive, and two batches were described as 'indeterminate'.

Where transmission of HIV in anti-D has occurred, it is quite possible that this contamination came from one blood donor; several batches may be contaminated because blood donations are pooled in order to make anti-D. This raises the question of whether pooling blood to make anti-D is truly essential to the manufacturing process, if this increases the chance of more women being infected.

As noted in Chapter 2, it is going to be impossible ever to give women complete assurance that they do not risk infection from a product of human origin. In response to the realization that HIV antibodies had been found in anti-D, Dumasia et al. (1989) stressed that 'pooled plasma should be free from any detectable infectious agent'. Here, the key word is 'detectable'. However sure we are that we have found a test for any potential virus, and the means to screen for and eradicate that virus from a product, we can never know all there is to know about virus detection and eradication. Does anybody really believe that we can conquer nature so completely? Furthermore, why aren't women being given information about the risks of viral contamination from anti-D in order to make the decision about this for themselves? Certain health practitioners may well believe that the benefits of anti-D outweigh the risks of viral contamination, but this is not their decision to make.

The controversy over the possibility that British blood supplies might be infected with new variant Creutzfeldt Jakob Disease (nvCJD) caused the British Government to announce in 1998 that the use of plasma collected from British donors was to be phased out; this would be replaced by foreign supplies. In a press release in May 1999, one pharmaceutical company (Baxter Healthcare Limited) announced that it was then in a position to import increased supplies of anti-D manufactured from plasma originating from North American donors. As previously discussed, the system of blood donation in the USA differs from that in the UK; donations of blood are paid for, which leads critics to question the motives of some donors and the potential quality of blood supplies.

Interestingly, the announcement that British blood is no longer used may be misleading without additional clarification; while British blood supplies are not currently being used in the manufacture of anti-D, they are still being used for other products. A number of scientists working in clinical blood transfusion confirmed in January 2000 that red cells, platelets and fresh frozen plasma are still manufactured from British blood. The blood itself is filtered and leuco-depleted – a process whereby the lymphocytes, or white blood cells, are removed, as it is thought that this is the part of blood which carries the nvCJD virus. While British women are not being given anti-D from this source, the question this raises is whether we yet know enough about nvCJD to be sure that this process is effective, or whether people receiving these other blood products from British sources remain at risk. It seems incredible that the British child-bearing woman is being offered a perceived degree of protection from nvCJD by being offered anti-D from foreign sources, yet if the same woman also required a blood transfusion she would be given British blood.

There has recently been a reduction in the number of people willing to become donors for the anti-D project because of the risk of virus transmission through blood (de Crespigny and Davison, 1995). These potential donors – who are rhesus negative – need to be given rhesus-positive red cells in order to cause the isoimmunization that would render them able to donate blood for the manufacture of anti-D. Their assessment of the risks of receiving blood products has led to their decision not to participate in the rhesus programme. When will all childbearing women be offered the chance to make the same assessment of risks to their health?

Without firm evidence of the quality of blood from any source, we can currently only offer women the information that there might be a small risk of viral transmission from anti-D. We have no accurate estimates of the frequency of this in practice. Admittedly this research would be expensive and lengthy, but the health of women and babies should be deemed more important than financial considerations.

Other risks of anti-D

Other aspects of the safety of anti-D have also been questioned: Ina May Gaskin, an American midwife, was one of the first to raise concerns about the effects of anti-D. She noticed the correlation between the issues in this area and the work of Durandy et al. (1981), who studied the effects of the administration of gamma globulin to children between the ages of 4 and 10 years. While the children did not show negative effects of this immediately, the researchers found that their immune systems were compromised for up to 5 months after receiving the gamma globulin. This not only supports the suggestion that women receiving postnatal anti-D may suffer effects to their immune system (Wickham, 1999b), but also raises the question of how much greater the effects of this would be on a developing baby, where anti-D is given antenatally (Gaskin, 1989).

Penni Harmon, another American midwife, looked at the risks and benefits of anti-D around the time that the American College of Obstetricians and Gynecologists were promoting the use of this in the antenatal period. While stressing the importance of maternal choice, she noted that 'the long-term risks {of anti-D} are not known, and there is controversy as to the safety of this application' (Harmon, 1987).

A less well-known risk of anti-D is that some forms contain the drug thimerosal, a mercury preservative which has been shown to cause severe allergic reactions and toxicity to humans. This is because thimerosal metabolizes as methylmercury, a substance that is toxic to humans – not least because, once ingested, it is not eliminated from the body. Thimerosal is also found in a number of vaccines given to children, and the World Health Organization raised concerns about this substance in 1990 (Vaccine Information and Awareness (VIA), personal correspondence, 1999). It is difficult to determine which forms of anti-D contain this drug, as this is not always printed on the product label. Consumer groups in the United States are campaigning for the removal of vaccines and other products containing thimerosal; they feel that the relevant governing bodies are not taking action on this issue, perhaps because of the massive cost implications of removing these products from use and replacing them with safer alternatives. Until then, it seems to be falling to individuals and groups to find out what the product they are being offered actually contains, and to campaign for alternatives to be made more widely available.

Measuring the effectiveness of the programme

A number of reviews of effectiveness of the rhesus prevention programme have been undertaken, which generally illustrate that there are still women who are not being offered anti-D at the appropriate points:

1. Tovey (1986) analysed 163 cases of maternal sensitization that occurred in the Yorkshire region between 1980 and 1983. He found that 36 of these cases were due to failures of administration, which means that these failures account for 22 per cent of the women who became sensitized.

2. Ghosh and Murphy (1994) studied all of the rhesus-negative women who completed a pregnancy in two Scottish regions in an 8-month period in 1992. This comprised 1120 women, 671 of whom gave birth to rhesus-positive babies. Their data showed failures at all stages of the programme; some women had no record of anti-D being offered or administered on their notes, only 69.6 per cent of women who had experienced an antenatal sensitizing event had been given anti-D, and one region was highlighted as failing to comply with the suggestion that postnatal anti-D should be offered routinely.

3. Of 922 rhesus-negative women whose care was audited in the Mersey area, a number experienced isoimmunization; Howard *et al.* (1997a) showed that 39 per cent of these sensitizations were a result of clinicians failing to follow the guidelines. Perhaps most significantly, only 19 of 24 women who experienced abdominal trauma were offered anti-D; most clinicians did not realize that this was a potentially sensitizing event.

4. Anti-D is not just an issue within midwifery and obstetric care; women who experience bleeding in early pregnancy, sometimes before they even know they are pregnant, may attend accident and emergency departments. Huggon and Watson's (1993) study highlighted serious problems with this aspect of the rhesus programme; this is discussed further in Chapter 4.

5. This problem is by no means unique to the United Kingdom; the American College of Obstetricians and Gynecologists (1999) also note cases of isoimmunization resulting from the failure of clinicians to offer anti-D to women.

Some of these reviews of clinicians' adherence to the recommendations appeared to result from researchers' acknowledgement of the twenty-fifth and thirtieth anniversaries of the introduction of anti-D, both of which occurred in the 1990s. The fact that, after this length of time, there are still a significant number of women who are not being offered this product ought to raise serious concerns among those who work with childbearing women. While it is imperative that women are enabled to make an informed choice about whether or not to have this product, surely all women who may be considered 'at risk' from potential isoimmunization ought to have the chance to receive anti-D if they so wish? Issues of effectiveness are also crucial in the debate concerning antenatal anti-D; these data are explored further in Chapter 4.

The problem of supply

Other researchers have questioned the routine use of anti-D in relation to the issue of supply; Australia, New Zealand and the UK have all experienced supply problems when production has failed to keep pace with demand (Horey, 1995). The issue of the UK now not using its own blood supplies can only exacerbate this problem. Indeed, the real cost of anti-D to the National Health Service has risen as a direct result of not using British blood as a source for anti-D. Previously, donated blood was sold to the companies who made anti-D, or traded in return for a discount on the product. If pharmaceutical companies are now buying blood from non-UK suppliers to make anti-D, then the Health Service is not receiving this cost benefit.

Research continues into other forms of anti-D, including monoclonal anti-D, which is still a blood product but is produced in a way that requires fewer donors. A cloning process is undertaken to replicate the active component of the anti-D, which is then introduced into a suitable medium for further development and transmission of the product. Following a clinical trial the use of monoclonal anti-D is permitted in Russia (Olovnikova et al., 1997), although this is not yet an option for clinical research in the UK (Saha, 1998). While the question of monoclonal anti-D raises many issues in itself, the fact that these possibilities continue to be pursued further confirms that issues relating to the supply of anti-D remain firmly on the European and global medical agenda.

In 1999, the American College of Obstetricians and Gynecologists expressed concern that overuse of anti-D may lead to a world-wide shortage of the product. While this is a fair point, it is interesting to note that this concern was raised by practitioners in one of the first countries to increase their need for anti-D dramatically by implementing the routine use of antenatal anti-D despite a relative lack of knowledge as to the risks and benefits of such a programme.

What information is currently available to women?

A brief survey of the information leaflets that may be offered to rhesus-negative women to inform them of the issues surrounding anti-D revealed the following general points:

- The vast majority of these leaflets are produced by the pharmaceutical companies that manufacture anti-D.
- The prime focus of the leaflets seems to be on explaining to rhesus-negative women why they need anti-D.
- The language used is simplistic and the leaflets are decorated with cute pictures of smiling babies and blood cells.
- The information given does not suggest that women need to make a choice in this area; the fact that all rhesus-negative women will need and accept anti-D appears to be a *fait accompli*.
- There is no mention of side effects in most of the leaflets.
- Where references to research are cited, the research is often that carried out internally by the pharmaceutical company. It is therefore impossible for women (or indeed their midwives) to obtain and verify.

During my research, I met with a representative of a pharmaceutical company that makes anti-D and we had a very interesting discussion about some of the issues. The most enlightening part of this discussion came when the representative asked me what I thought of their patient {sic} information literature. I shared my own opinions and thoughts on this with him, and then asked him whether they had piloted the leaflets with a group of women, or asked women what it was that they wanted to know about anti-D. The idea was obviously a new one to him, although I am pleased to say he gave it due consideration and thought it was worth following up. I must stress that this was a very pleasant man, who I felt truly cared about women, and I didn't imagine that he would knowingly do anything to hurt or misinform women. However, even paternalism in the shape of doting grandfathers is still paternalism. Could it be that the industry in which he works is so out of touch with the users of their product that they do not even think to discuss whether the information the users receive is beneficial to them?

Saha, a British obstetrician, raised questions about women's involvement in the rhesus programme in a letter to the *British Medical Journal* (Saha, 1988). She conducted an *ad hoc* survey of 12 rhesus-negative women who had received or been offered anti-D, and found that not one of them knew that anti-D was a blood product. They had assumed that it was either synthetic or from another natural source. Saha suggests it is imperative that women are counselled about the source of anti-D and the possibility of acquiring blood-borne infections.

Following the publication of Saha's letter, I conducted my own *ad hoc* survey of eight obstetricians; not one of them made efforts to ensure that women received this information in practice, and all but one felt that women should not be made to worry about such issues. The general feeling was that anti-D was vital to women, and therefore women should not 'worry themselves' about the minuscule risk of infection. Midwives were more likely to talk to women about anti-D as an option, but, anecdotally, those working in hospitals seem to be less likely to offer an explicit choice or to possess the knowledge base to support discussion with women on the issue. There could be many reasons for this, not least the pressure felt by midwives from strict policies they are expected to follow.

What issues remain?

There continues to be a lack of what could be described as 'woman-centred' research into anti-D. Pharmaceutical companies continue to fund much of the research concerning anti-D. While this may be normal in the industry, it is worth reflecting on how appropriate this is. Some of the authors who have been involved in anti-D research for years have openly stated their sources of funding, while others have left this aspect of their research open to question. It would be interesting to know just what percentage of the trials and other research has been funded by pharmaceutical companies.

It is clear from all sources that rhesus disease remains a problem, although so far nobody has managed to determine accurately why this is the case. In a 1997 *British Medical Journal* editorial, van Dijk suggested that one of the reasons concerned the problem of health professionals not following guidelines which state that they need to offer anti-D to women 'at risk' (van Dijk, 1997). As above, this is clearly an important issue, and one that must be addressed sooner rather than later. Van Dijk adds that 'pregnant women ... should be educated about the condition, so that they recognize the need for treatment should a sensitizing event occur' (van Dijk, 1997). Perhaps this is an unfortunate use of terminology, but it may illustrate the trend where, even in the late 1990s, doctors feel the need to seek compliance from women rather than working in partnership to enable informed decision-making.

It is also clear that women should be offered the appropriate information, and if health professionals are unable to implement the guidelines by offering anti-D to the women who may benefit from this, it would seem sensible for women to take the lead in this instance. However, rather than educating women for compliance, current Government policy (the Cumberledge Report, 1993) suggests that:

> The woman must be the focus of maternity care. She should be able to feel that she is in control of what is happening to her and able to make decisions about her care, based on her needs, having discussed matters fully with the professionals involved.

The recommendation that women should be fully informed and involved in the choice of whether or not they receive anti-D in the postnatal and/or antenatal periods is not being fully implemented in practice. The importance of giving up-to-date and full information to rhesus-negative women cannot be over stressed, and is a fundamental first step in the movement towards a more woman-centred approach to the rhesus programme.

CHAPTER FOUR

The question of antenatal anti-D

While the initial recommendations for the administration of anti-D concerned the immediate postnatal period (that is, within 72 hours of the birth of a rhesus-positive baby), these were soon extended to include potential sensitizing events in the antenatal period (see Chapter 2). If a woman experienced vaginal bleeding or any kind of trauma to the uterus, placenta or umbilical cord, the potential for transplacental haemorrhage existed and she would therefore be offered anti-D to prevent the development of antibodies and iso-immunization.

It seems sensible and appropriate to offer women this option where there is evidence of actual or potential fetomaternal transfusion, although it has been suggested that not all transplacental haemorrhage in pregnancy can be predicted. Transplacental haemorrhage that occurs in the absence of clinical signs is termed 'silent', and the existence of this phenomenon forms part of the basis for the suggestion that anti-D should be routinely given to all rhesus-negative women at set times during the antenatal period to protect against this possibility.

This suggestion is controversial, and there has been much debate in the midwifery and medical literature concerning the advantages and disadvantages of such a policy. This chapter will explore some of those arguments, and consider the research that has been undertaken in this area. The debate surrounding the routine administration of anti-D during pregnancy began in 1967, with the suggestion by Zipursky and Israels that consideration of antenatal administration may reduce the rate of sensitization. Bowman and Pollock (1978) followed this up with the specific recommendation that anti-D should be administered to all rhesus-negative women at 28 weeks to prevent sensitization in pregnancy. This appears to be the first specific reference to a suggested antenatal anti-D protocol in the literature, and was made by a researcher who works with a Canadian pharmaceutical laboratory.

The debate continued throughout the 1980s, and British researchers were divided between those who saw antenatal anti-D as a wholly beneficial intervention that would save babies, and those who urged caution for a variety of reasons. This intervention is now used routinely in some countries, including the USA, where in 1983 the American College of Obstetricians and Gynecologists recommended the routine use of antenatal anti-D at 28 weeks of pregnancy. Germany has also had an antenatal anti-D protocol since 1990 (Schlensker and Kruger, 1996), although the UK has thus far resisted such a programme. However, this situation may be about to change; a consensus conference in 1997 decided to recommend routine antenatal administration in the UK, and the issue is currently being debated on practical, professional and political levels.

The case for antenatal anti-D

A number of researchers have called for a policy of routine administration of anti-D in the antenatal period; citing evidence that the administration of postnatal anti-D does not prevent all cases of isoimmunization, they feel that routine antenatal administration is the best way forward in moving closer to 100 per cent protection from isoimmunization. The following studies are representative of the data presented in this area in support of the argument for routine antenatal anti-D.

- Hughes *et al.* (1994) carried out research in Scotland, looking retrospectively at 80 babies with rhesus disease who were born between 1985 and 1990. Data were available to categorize the cause of isoimmunization in 70 of these pregnancies, and it was found that seven cases were due to isoimmunization before 1970 (i.e. before anti-D was available), 10 to clinicians' failure to implement the programme, and the other 53 to the failure of the current guidelines to protect against isoimmunization. They suggest that antenatal administration would have prevented many of these women from being isoimmunized.

- Derbyshire is one of the areas in the UK where women having their first baby are already offered antenatal anti-D at 28 and 34 weeks of pregnancy, and Mayne et al. (1997) assessed the effectiveness of this programme. They showed a fall in the mean overall sensitization rate from 1.12 per cent in 1988–1991 (before the onset of the antenatal programme) to 0.28 per cent in 1993–1995. They also noted that one of the benefits of the programme was an increase in requests from women for anti-D in response to potential sensitizing events in pregnancy. While they suggest that this was probably the result of heightened awareness, they do not offer any insight into what difference this would have made to the actual sensitization rates. While it is certainly unlikely that it would have decreased the sensitization rates by quite the same amount that routine antenatal anti-D did, it may well have made some difference by ensuring that more of the women experiencing sensitizing events were offered anti-D. Other studies have shown that non-compliance by clinicians is a factor in antenatal sensitization rates; research looking into the effectiveness of raising consumer and professional awareness alongside the administration of routine antenatal anti-D would have reduced the potential for confounding variables and offered more insight into the real effects of this as an intervention.

- The following year, McSweeney et al. (1998) published the results of a study carried out in Yorkshire in which they looked back at women's medical notes. Although they found that professionals failed to offer anti-D in 48 per cent of cases where women experienced potential sensitizing events in the antenatal period, they advocated the use of routine antenatal anti-D in order to cover the other instances of isoimmunization. Their estimate is that at least 86 per cent of the cases where women became isoimmunized were preventable by antenatal anti-D administration, although this is a higher figure than in some of the other studies. They do, however, raise a number of other questions, including that of appropriate dosage, which may impact on their data.

Some of these studies (and many of the others carried out in this area) are retrospective; that is, they look back on events that have already occurred in order to attempt to extrapolate meaningful data for the future. However, the data gathered in a retrospective study are regarded by researchers as less meaningful than prospective (forward-looking) research, where there is less potential for bias. The use of women's case notes in such research can bring problems; many aspects of care are not always well documented by professionals, and this can lead to bias in the results of the study. For instance, if a clinician did not document the occurrence of a potentially sensitizing event, or perhaps failed to ask the woman about these, then it would look as if the woman had experienced silent fetomaternal haemorrhage if she then became isoimmunized. Some of the studies do not give enough information to enable the reader to critique the study effectively and judge for themselves the quality of the research. For example, there may be no details of the events considered as potentially sensitizing, and the quality of information given in the women's notes may be inadequate.

Much of the evidence cited in this area, although interesting and useful in other ways, does not look at the effectiveness of antenatal anti-D in the light of prospective, randomized controlled trials. Because of this, reviewers from the Cochrane database (Crowther and Kierse, 1999) look for examples of those clinical trials that meet specific quality criteria for use in their reviews of the evidence in a particular area. Reviewers potentially have access to more information than is given in published papers of a particular study, and it may then be considered that only those trials included in the review are of a high enough standard to be considered 'sound' in terms of quantitative research evidence.

Of the antenatal anti-D trials conducted, only two are considered by these reviewers to reach the standard for inclusion. One of these (Lee and Rawlinson, 1995) gave women in the treatment group two doses of 50 mg (250 iu) of anti-D at 28 and 34 weeks, and showed no statistically significant difference between their outcomes and those of women in the group who had not received antenatal anti-D. However, researchers in the study by Huchet et al. (1987) gave a larger dose of anti-D (500 iu) at 28 and 34 weeks and showed a clear reduction in the incidence of isoimmunization at between 2 and 12 months, although no data regarding subsequent pregnancy in those women were available. The reviewers concluded that there was still a need for consideration of other issues, such as cost and supply of anti-D.

Both of these studies were randomized, although neither was single- or double-blinded; again, the question of whether bias could have entered in this way needs to be raised. Data were also lost for a proportion of women in each trial; 4.3 per cent of the women in the Huchet *et al.* (1987) trial and 22 per cent of the women in the Lee and Rawlinson (1995) trial did not have their data included in the results because they were 'lost to follow-up', and again this may have impacted on the results. Both trials included only women who were pregnant for the first time or who were having their first term baby (perhaps following a previous miscarriage or abortion). Crowther and Kierse (1999) conclude that further research is needed to determine the dosage, timing and number of treatments in an antenatal programme, and also raise questions regarding the cost-effectiveness of routine antenatal administration.

Thus, while research supporting the routine antenatal administration of anti-D is widely available, the quality of some of the evidence may be lacking. Those who look closely at such research may agree that there is really only one trial of any quality that shows this to be effective. Of course, just as with postnatal anti-D, the fact that this trial shows anti-D to be effective certainly does not mean it is necessary or beneficial for all women; this is another issue entirely.

The case for caution

There is a great deal of debate among researchers and clinicians regarding antenatal anti-D; the fact that even those who share a common philosophy cannot agree on this issue (although there is certainly a general consensus regarding postnatal anti-D) illustrates the level of controversy that still remains in this area. While the argument put forward in favour of routine antenatal anti-D is relatively simple – that this will prevent those few cases of isoimmunization that occur despite routine postnatal administration – there are three main arguments against this. The first of these concerns the difficulty in trying to establish how effective antenatal anti-D would be when there are still questions and problems regarding the current programme of routine postnatal administration and antenatal administration in response to a potentially sensitizing event. The second concerns the potential risks of antenatal administration to women and their unborn babies, while the third concerns the costs of such a programme.

How effective is anti-D?

A number of researchers have considered the subject of antenatal anti-D in relation to the evidence surrounding the current guidelines for the administration of this product. As discussed in Chapter 3, Ghosh and Murphy's (1994) Scottish study showed that just over 30 per cent of women who had experienced an antenatal sensitizing event had not been offered anti-D. Clearly, it is not helpful to begin an antenatal programme if a proportion of the women who are becoming sensitized during pregnancy are doing so as a result of professional failure to offer anti-D after a potentially sensitizing event. Rather than subjecting all women to antenatal anti-D because some clinicians fail to offer this to the women that really need it, we need to consider how this trend can be reversed. We also need to establish how many women are becoming sensitized as a result of failure to implement the current guidelines, and not include these women in figures that are being used to promote the uptake of routine antenatal prophylaxis.

Howard *et al.* (1997a) are among those who propose that closer adherence to the 1991 recommendations might further reduce the incidence of isoimmunization. They suggest that we should evaluate the effect of applying the recommendations more carefully before implementing routine antenatal prophylaxis or considering the use of higher doses of anti-D. These researchers examined the notes of 922 women who gave birth in seven hospitals, and found that only 20 per cent of women who had experienced abdominal trauma had been offered anti-D. They also identified problems with professionals' understanding of the appropriate doses in pregnancy. Both of these failures are likely to lead to an increase in sensitization, which clearly cannot be attributed to 'silent' events. This study also reported only 95 per cent adherence to the recommendation to offer women postnatal anti-D; medical notes relating to women who did not receive anti-D did not record that these women declined this, which leads to the assumption that it was simply overlooked by clinicians.

Another British study that considered adherence to the guidelines for administering anti-D after sensitizing events in pregnancy was conducted by Huggon and Watson (1993). This study was carried out in the accident and emergency department, and focused on 29 women who arrived following a threatened miscarriage. Theoretically, these women should have had their blood group determined and, if they were found to be rhesus negative, should have been offered anti-D. The researchers found that only eight women were tested to establish their blood group, and none of those women who were rhesus negative were offered anti-D.

Following this small-scale study, a larger review of accident and emergency departments in the UK was carried out by Gilling-Smith *et al.* (1997). Of the 88 accident and emergency units that dealt with women who experienced bleeding in early pregnancy, only 23 per cent administered anti-D when this was appropriate. There were other worrying statistics; only 84 per cent of the units could actually obtain anti-D, while 37 per cent did not have access to Kleihauer testing to determine whether a woman had experienced a larger bleed than would be covered by the standard dose.

These results are a reminder of the fact that it is not only those working in midwifery and obstetrics who need to be aware of the issues. If staff in accident and emergency departments are not aware of the need to offer anti-D, then perhaps women who experience bleeding in early pregnancy should be advised to go elsewhere. The implications for the antenatal anti-D debate are equally clear; if 77 per cent of accident and emergency departments are not offering anti-D to women who have knowingly experienced a sensitizing event, then how far would reversal of this trend impact on the figures relating to antenatal sensitization? Do midwives meeting women for the first time in pregnancy routinely check whether rhesus-negative women have already experienced bleeding and whether they have been offered anti-D as a result? Again, it is difficult to draw conclusions because so many of the studies in this area are retrospective and consequently flawed by the failure of attendants to include the relevant details in women's notes; there are, however, questions that would seem to warrant fairly rapid answers.

Tovey (1986) showed that 22 per cent of the women in his study became sensitized as a result of 'failure of administration'. While he suggests that antenatal administration of anti-D may have protected 40 per cent of the women who became sensitized during the period of his study, we need to examine carefully what these figures mean in reality. While 40 per cent appears to be a relatively large proportion of women, we must remember that this is not 40 per cent of rhesus-negative women or even 40 per cent of women who are 'at risk', but rather 40 per cent of the women who actually became sensitized. This group is a tiny proportion of the rhesus-negative women who became pregnant and gave birth in the 3-year period studied, and the accuracy of these figures is vitally important when considering the risks as well as the benefits of this kind of programme.

A more helpful perspective on this issue is that offered by Robson *et al.* (1998), who reported the consensus conference's estimate that between 2500 and 3000 women need to be given antenatal anti-D in order to prevent one death from rhesus haemolytic disease. (In reality the number of women may be even higher than this, as discussed below.) Again, we are looking at the issues on a population basis, which may not be useful for individuals. A more helpful statistic for women deciding whether or not to have routine antenatal anti-D would be that which concerned their chance of experiencing antenatal sensitization in the absence of clinical factors (e.g. trauma to the abdomen or amniocentesis). However, it has proved impossible to extract an accurate estimate of this figure due to the lack of sound data available.

The concern that the vast majority of the women receiving antenatal anti-D do not need or benefit from this is illustrated in part by the fact that around 40 per cent of those women have rhesus-negative babies, and so are not in any danger from transplacental bleeding. While research is being conducted into whether it is possible to determine the blood group of a baby before it is born (Armstrong-Fisher *et al.*, 1998; Miller *et al.*, 1998), the only way of predicting this at the present time is to determine the blood type of the baby's father. If he is rhesus negative, then all of the couple's babies will be rhesus negative. If he is rhesus positive and found to be heterozygous there is a chance the baby will be rhesus negative, but if he is homozygous rhesus positive then all of the couple's babies will be rhesus positive.

Should the paternal blood testing that would provide this kind of information be made available to women who would prefer to take this step before consenting to the administration of anti-D? It has never been suggested that women who give birth to a rhesus-negative baby should receive anti-D in the postnatal period, so why should women not have the option of finding out whether they are part of the 40 per cent who do not need anti-D at all? Does the cost of paternal blood testing really exceed the cost of administering two doses of antenatal anti-D? The costs of these two options are not only monetary; there are negligible potential side effects to paternal blood testing, whereas the potential cost of antenatal anti-D to the health of women and babies may be significant (see below).

It should also be noted that women who are pregnant with their last child will not benefit from antenatal anti-D. Even so, it is not routine practice to discuss this with women in relation to their personal need for anti-D. Some members of the medical profession may feel they have good reason for not including this option, in that a few women may change their minds about this, perhaps deciding to have another baby if they take a new partner or suffer the loss of other children. Surely it is unreasonably paternalistic to make this decision for all women, some of whom may be very sure about their choice or unable to have further babies for other reasons? There must be ways of ensuring that women are clearly informed of all of the potential outcomes and options, while enabling them to make this decision for themselves.

Potential risks of antenatal anti-D

It was noted in Chapter 1 that anti-D is a drug that is given to a person who does not physically benefit, perhaps to the detriment of their health, in order to benefit another who does not yet exist. When anti-D is administered in pregnancy, this drug may additionally cause risk to another person whom it does not benefit, the unborn child, in order to offer protection to the child's potential future siblings. The fact that there has been no research investigating the effects of anti-D on the unborn child is one of the factors of concern to those currently calling for caution (Gaskin, 1989; Coombes, 1999). This is not only in hypothetical terms; Gaskin's work does point to several potential risk factors where babies are exposed to anti-D, including immune system compromise and potential problems during later reproduction for rhesus-negative baby girls exposed to anti-D *in utero*.

Two further potential risks of antenatal anti-D are discussed in the medical literature, although this does not mean that these are the only possible risks; there may be others that have not as yet been predicted. The first risk is that of augmentation, or enhanced anti-D immunization (Urbaniak, 1998). This describes the situation where a woman who is given passive anti-D during the antenatal period could, upon exposure to rhesus-positive cells (via transplacental haemorrhage) mount a primary immune response to these. This is the exact opposite to what anti-D is intended to do, and has been observed in experimental models (Pollack *et al.*, 1968). Urbaniak (1998) notes that 'the experimental data {relating to this} in immunized volunteers are conflicting', which would seem suggestive of a need for further study.

The second concern is the effect of passive anti-D on the unborn baby. Although Gaskin's evidence concerning immune system compromise does not seem to have been heeded by the medical profession in general, other risks to the baby have been discussed. Some of these concern the fact that about 10 per cent of the anti-D given to the mother will cross the placenta to the baby (Hughes-Jones *et al.*, 1971; Urbaniak, 1998). Studies have shown that this causes a proportion of babies to test positive for antiglobulins (via a direct Coombs test) after they are born (Bowman and Pollock, 1978; Tovey *et al.*, 1983; Herman *et al.*, 1984). The few studies that have looked at this have suggested that, while babies may suffer some anaemia, this does not require treatment in the immediate postnatal period. Although Romm (1999) points out that the manufacturers of anti-D clearly state that this should not be given to babies, nobody has considered the question of whether there are long-term consequences of this. It should be remembered that unborn babies will also be exposed to the risks that women face, such as that of virus transmission. Is it also possible that a baby could suffer the equivalent of an anaphylactic reaction? If this is a possibility, how would this manifest, and is there any way we would be able to treat this before it was too late?

The fact that there is little evidence regarding these risks does not necessarily mean that they exist only in theory; while it is true that there is currently only a small amount of specific evidence relating to this, it is also true that there is no guarantee of safety. There has been no systematic study that looks at the short- and long-term side effects of anti-D in babies (Urbaniak, 1998). If research is not undertaken into the potential risks to babies, then the very programme that leads to the administration of anti-D to all rhesus-negative pregnant women will also experiment with the health of their babies. Having said this, if the programme is treated in the same way as the original programme of postnatal anti-D administration, then we will not be seeing studies to assess the relative safety of this product, and so may never find out whether babies are suffering as a result.

How will we find out what the effects of anti-D on unborn babies are? We may notice a new variation on a childhood disease in a few years time, or that the health of children is deteriorating further, but without effective ways of measuring the risks of the rhesus programme we will have no idea whether this is the cause of such problems or whether it is safe for the majority of unborn babies. This can only be exacerbated by the fact that we do not know what the optimal dose of antenatal anti-D is; we may be exposing women and babies to more of this product than they need.

Issues of cost

The third argument against the routine administration of antenatal anti-D concerns the cost of such a programme. At the time of publishing, the cost of a 500-iu vial of anti-D is £18. The cost of the equipment needed to administer this (needle, water, syringe, cotton wool and so on) is roughly £0.15 per injection, while the cost of staff time has been estimated to be £3.33 per administration (that is, 10 minutes of a midwife's time where the total cost of that midwife is £20 per hour). This brings the rough average cost of administering a 500-iu dose of anti-D to £21.50. Multiply this by the 60 000 British women who receive postnatal anti-D every year, and the first part of the bill comes to around £1.29 million per year. (This does not include the administration of extra postnatal doses of anti-D for women who require this, nor does it include any estimate of accidental spoiling of product or breakage of equipment.)

If routine antenatal administration were adopted, the majority of the 100 000 rhesus-negative women who give birth in the UK each year would be offered it. The Royal College of Obstetricians and Gynaecologists suggest administering this twice during pregnancy, which brings the bill for routine antenatal administration to £4.3 million per year in the UK, and the total cost to £5.59 million per year for the standard doses alone. Again, the actual cost would be higher than this once further postnatal doses and those offered following sensitizing events were taken into account.

Around £1.72 million of this total would be spent on administering antenatal anti-D to women with rhesus-positive babies. Does the evidence for antenatal anti-D really justify increasing the cost of routine administration more than fourfold rather than funding research that might help determine which women really need this and whether antenatal isoimmunization can be predicted? Of course, issues of finance should be secondary to risks to women and babies, but looking at the actual cost (which will almost inevitably be higher than that estimated here) may put the issues more into perspective.

When discussing the issue of how many women need to be given anti-D to save one baby, it would seem pertinent to use the data offered by Whitfield *et al.* (1997), which offer the most pessimistic estimates. These data suggest that there is serious underestimation of deaths from rhesus disease, and that these may number up to 50 cases a year in the UK rather than the average of nine or ten which are reported as such (Clarke and Hussey, 1994). Some of these babies are lost due to miscarriage in early pregnancy, while others will survive beyond the first week in which neonatal deaths are calculated. Some of these babies' mothers will have become isoimmunized not through silent fetomaternal haemorrhage but because of clinicians' failure to offer anti-D at the appropriate times, but approximately half of these deaths are thought to be preventable by antenatal anti-D (van Dijk, 1997).

Around 100 000 rhesus-negative women give birth in the UK every year. This means that somewhere in the region of 4000 women (and their unborn babies) need to be given antenatal anti-D in order to save one baby. (This differs from the previously discussed estimate of 2500–3000, which was presented by Robson *et al.* (1998), but as neither this paper nor the proceedings of the consensus conference where it was discussed showed how this figure was calculated, it is impossible to determine where the discrepancy lies.) To put it another way, any given woman has a 1 in 4000 chance of losing a subsequent baby from rhesus disease if she does not have routine antenatal anti-D. This does not, of course, mean that antenatal anti-D will offer her total protection against this outcome, just as the current postnatal programme offers no absolute guarantee. Is it really so outrageous to be calling for more research into which women might really benefit from antenatal anti-D rather than giving this to 3999 women and unborn babies unnecessarily in order to save one baby?

It is important to acknowledge that not all babies suffering from rhesus disease die as a result; some will survive, although those with severe forms of this will require intensive care, another issue that affects costs. Unfortunately, those who offer cost analyses in this area do not usually show how they perform their calculations or reach their conclusions; we are often asked to accept their findings without seeing the actual sums. This fact forced me to make my own broad estimates of the costs of an antenatal anti-D programme.

Those who call for caution in relation to antenatal anti-D are not able accurately to compare the health costs of isoimmunization with the health costs of the routine administration of anti-D because trials which have specifically looked for the problems potentially caused by this do not exist. In any case, how can the situation of women with compromised immune systems be compared with that of women who face the levels of intervention offered in pregnancies complicated by rhesus disease? Or the situation of babies who have suffered *in utero* or as a result of their mothers receiving anti-D with that of babies who spend their early weeks in neonatal care units? There is no easy way to analyse these data.

It would seem that these situations are incomparable, and that the only people who can make the decision regarding anti-D are the individual women. This would suggest that, even if antenatal anti-D becomes available on the strength of the evidence presented to those with the power to make such decisions, this should not be considered a routine intervention but rather an option offered to women. The proviso should be that the evidence must be freely available to women so that they can make their decisions based on a fair appraisal of this, rather than being swayed by hospital information leaflets advising them only of the benefits of this procedure or by professionals who are biased in their opinions.

Debating the issues

In 1997, a consensus conference was held so that a group of experts could determine a national recommendation in the area of antenatal anti-D administration. These experts gathered to assess the evidence, including much of that presented here, and make recommendations to the Royal College of Obstetricians and Gynaecologists and the Royal College of Physicians of Edinburgh. While the term 'conference' suggests a large number of experts, in fact only 12 were included in the decision-making process. This group, which was said to include a 'range of perspectives'

(Urbaniak, 1988), included haematologists, obstetricians, general practitioners and even a medical journalist. Significantly, a number of groups were not represented; no consumer-focused childbirth organizations or childbearing women were invited for their opinions, and there was no clinical midwifery representation on the group. This seems extremely undemocratic, as it is women who receive the product and usually midwives who inform them of the issues and administer it.

Yet again, groups of predominantly male doctors felt able to make decisions about women's health and choices without consulting the women themselves. Perhaps this is because it was perceived that lay women and consumer organizations would not understand the issues; anti-D is a complex subject and the research could be seen as unapproachable by some. In response to this, of the more than 100 'lay' women interviewed about anti-D during the course of my research, not one failed to understand the issues. The same goes for representatives of consumer organizations. Indeed, it is apparent that a proportion of the women who face this kind of decision spend so much time doing their own research in order to understand the issues that they often end up knowing more about it than their caregivers. Maybe the real reason women were not invited to participate in this decision-making process is that doctors still fail to perceive women as the focus of maternity care.

The conference itself resulted in the publication of the recommendations concerning antenatal anti-D; the group decided that (Urbaniak, 1998):

> Because all RhD negative pregnant women are at risk from hidden bleeds, they should be given anti-D IgG prophylactically.

Some of the issues raised in the proceedings of this conference may be worthy of closer attention:

- In relation to current failures of implementation, the conference noted their concern that 'there is abundant evidence that the recommendations are not being fully applied' (Urbaniak, 1998). They did not, however, feel that this issue warranted further investigation before making the decision to recommend routine antenatal anti-D.

- The conference recommended that 'the viral and other safety issues raised by changes in product manufacture are kept under rigorous review' (Urbaniak, 1998). However, the recommendations include no suggestions as to how this should be carried out or who should be responsible for such reviews.

- Another recommendation concerned the suggestion that 'information leaflets concerning the recommendations should be given to RhD negative women and their partners'. This may be an issue which the midwifery profession needs to debate in relation to informed choice and the need for balanced information; as discussed in Chapter 2, the information leaflets currently available are biased towards women's acceptance of anti-D rather than the facilitation of informed choice.

A number of organizations have responded to these conclusions, which have caused some considerable concern to those who work closely with childbearing women. The Royal College of Midwives is lobbying the Department of Health to put the new suggestions before the National Institute for Clinical Excellence (NICE) for review before the guidelines are accepted nationally (Royal College of Midwives, 1999). To date, this body has not indicated if or when the recommendations will be considered.

In 1999, the United Kingdom Central Council for Nurses Midwives and Health Visitors also raised concerns about the guidelines advocating the use of anti-D in the antenatal period (Coombes, 1999). They raised the issue of the lack of testing of the product for routine use, and reiterated that there was no sound evidence to suggest that antenatal administration was beneficial. They also highlighted the fact that around 40 per cent of the 100 000 or so women who would receive antenatal anti-D each year in the UK would be carrying rhesus-negative babies, and therefore would have received this unnecessarily. Consumer and midwifery organizations are equally concerned that women should be able to make choices based on the evidence available, rather than the opinions of a group of people who may have a different philosophy from that of the women directly affected.

Midwifery evidence

The debate regarding antenatal anti-D might be informed by the findings discussed in the next few chapters. The issues that arose from my own research included the possibility that women might be able to take measures to optimize the strength of their placenta and thus protect themselves and their babies from fetomaternal haemorrhage. This is discussed further in Chapter 9. Other findings included the suggestion that we may need to broaden the list of interventions that may give rise to fetomaternal haemorrhage; Chapter 7 outlines the midwives' suggestions that antenatal interventions such as ultrasonography may give rise to transplacental haemorrhage in some women.

This does not necessarily mean that women need to be offered anti-D following such interventions; another possibility is that some women may want to reconsider their need for this kind of procedure in the light of this evidence. It may be that the women who choose to have ultrasonography and similar interventions in pregnancy are the women who also experience silent fetomaternal haemorrhage; research may help to determine which women experience this silent fetomaternal haemorrhage and whether it is always as 'silent' as is currently thought.

CHAPTER FIVE

The search for midwifery evidence

Analysis of the existing research in the area of routine anti-D administration suggested that there were a number of areas that appeared promising in terms of starting points for debate, discussion and further research. One of the most noticeable features of the body of evidence surrounding anti-D was that no research had been undertaken by midwives, or within a midwifery framework. It may be for this reason that interpretations of the research have, to date, focused on the need to give anti-D to all women, rather than considering the data supporting the theory that anti-D may not be necessary on a routine basis. For all of these reasons I chose to explore this issue further, from the perspective of the 'midwifery model', in the hope that some of the gaps in our knowledge as highlighted in the previous chapters may be filled by other types of evidence.

It soon became apparent that it was necessary to focus in on one aspect of anti-D administration; to consider both postnatal and antenatal administration within a primary research study was going to be both unwieldy and potentially confusing. The choice was therefore made to consider only the routine postnatal administration of anti-D. This could be seen as the 'baseline' routine intervention in the area and, consequently, constitutes the most obvious starting point for such research. It was of course possible that data could be extrapolated in relation to other areas of the anti-D debate, or discussion encouraged, although this was not a primary aim of the study.

On reading the original research concerning postnatal anti-D, it became clear that it was characterized by three main features:

1. Although postnatal anti-D was proven effective on a population basis, the research also showed that not all of the women in the control groups developed rhesus antibodies. This provided a basis of support for the proposition that anti-D may not be necessary as a routine postnatal intervention, although no further evidence was available as to which women may not need this product to prevent isoimmunization.

2. The research had all been carried out within a quantitative, medical and scientific paradigm, through randomized clinical trials. No midwives were involved in these trials, and no work was undertaken within a 'midwifery model'. The implication of this is that there may be other knowledge, held by midwives and within this midwifery model, that may inform the subject area for others.

3. Inevitably, the focus of these clinical trials was on gaining evidence for use on a population level; consequently, little evidence is available to assist individual women in making an informed decision in this area. However, while this enables policy-makers to base their guidelines upon population statistics and financial implications, women are individuals, and need more and varied evidence on which they can base their decisions, while taking their own circumstances and beliefs into account.

I began discussing the subject with midwifery colleagues, and started a dialogue with midwives and women who used the Internet to discuss such issues; this was partially triggered by experience with women in practice, which led to the discovery of a source of alternative viewpoints (Wickham, 1999a). These viewpoints did not all agree with the medical interpretations, and it became evident that midwives may have as yet untapped knowledge, beliefs and experiences in this area which might expand the debate and the evidence, while also acting as a trigger for further research. This led to the decision to undertake research with midwives and within the midwifery model, where evidence may be gathered from a number of sources, including knowledge gathered from experience, world view and reflection upon an area of practice.

The midwifery and medical models

As the theoretical framework of this study involves consideration of the 'medical' and 'midwifery' models in their approach to the childbearing process, it may be appropriate to define these at this stage. The terms 'midwifery model' and 'medical model', although used in everyday conversation by practitioners, may not have universal meanings. The main themes of the models as used here are outlined below; Table 5.1 provides an initial overview of the area, although this necessarily defines the extremes of the models. The philosophy of many practitioners may fall somewhere in between these reference points. It should also be stressed that not all midwives practise within the midwifery model, and neither do all doctors accept the medical model; there is a certain amount of crossover, and the models relate primarily to philosophical standpoints rather than absolute professional stances.

Table 5.1 Aspects of the medical and midwifery models

Aspect of approach	Medical model	Midwifery model
General view of childbearing	Inherently risky, abnormal	Normal life event/rite of passage, occasionally deviates from the norm
Focus of care	Safety, physical factors and measurements	Woman's defined, holistic needs
System of care	Usually hospital-based; routinization/ standardization of care may occur	Usually community/home based; care geared to individual needs
Dominant emotions	Fear	Trust, respect for nature
Basis of evidence informing practice	Quantitative controlled trials, positivist methodology; proof	Qualitative, experiential, intuitive knowledge

This area has been further explored by Davis-Floyd (1992), who built upon the work of several theorists to produce a comparison of the technocratic and holistic models of birth. These differ from original definitions and conceptualizations of the medical and midwifery models in that they describe the 'bigger picture' of attitudes towards birth on a systemic level. The aspects of her models that are relevant here are outlined in Table 5.2.

Table 5.2 The technocratic and wholistic models of birth (adapted from Davis-Floyd, 1992)

The technocratic model of birth	*The wholistic model of birth*
Male perspective	Female perspective
Male-centred	Female-centred
Woman = object	Woman = subject
Female = defective male	Female normal in own terms
Classifying, separating approach	Holistic, integrating approach
Mind is above, separate from body	Mind and body are one
Body = machine	Body = organism
Female body = defective machine	Female body = healthy organism
Pregnancy/birth inherently pathological	Pregnancy/birth inherently normal
Doctor = technician	Midwife = nurturer
Hospital = factory	Home = nurturing environment
Baby = product	Baby and mother inseparable unit
Fetus is separate from mother	Baby and mother are one
Safety of fetus pitted against emotional needs of mother	Intimate connection between growth of baby and state of mother
Interests of mother/baby antagonistic	Good for mother = good for child
Supremacy of technology	Sufficiency of nature
Importance of science, things	Importance of people
Action based on facts, measurements	Action based on body knowledge, intuition
Only technical knowledge valued	Experiential, emotional knowledge valued as highly as technical knowledge
Responsibility is the doctor's	Responsibility is the mother's
The doctor delivers the baby	The mother births the baby

Midwives around the world are now calling for more support of the midwifery (or wholistic) model of birth, primarily because they believe this to form a more accurate representation of 'the way birth is'. Bryar (1988) argues that, in recent years, midwifery has been undertaken within an obstetric or medical model, and finds a great need for midwifery models in order to redress the balance that has been tipped towards the potentially pathological. In 1992, the Midwives' Alliance of North America (MANA) set out to encapsulate the values, ethics and principles which they felt to be important in the relationship between midwife and mother. Their statement, shown in Table 5.3, also forms an important view of what has become known as the midwifery model of birth.

Table 5.3 MANA statement of values and ethics (Midwives' Alliance of North America, 1998)

We value:

- The oneness of the pregnant mother and her unborn child; an inseparable and interdependent whole.
- The essential mystery of birth.
- Pregnancy and birth as natural processes that science will never supplant.
- The integrity of life's experiences; the physical, emotional, mental, psychological and spiritual components of a process are inseparable.
- Pregnancy and birth as intimate, internal, sexual and private events to be shared in the environment and with the attendants a woman chooses.
- A mother's intuitive knowledge of herself and her baby before and after birth.
- A woman's innate ability to nurture her pregnancy and birth her baby; the power and beauty of her body as it grows and the awesome strength summoned in labor.
- Our relationship to a process larger than ourselves, recognizing that birth is something we can seek to learn from and know, but never control.
- The concept of self-responsibility and the right of individuals to make choices regarding what they deem best for themselves.

Although midwives vary in their individual beliefs and values, these examples describe what is generally understood by the midwifery model, and the differences between this and the medical model of birth. This model is accepted and utilized by the participants, and forms the basis of the paradigm which has been developed.

Having determined the theoretical framework upon which research would be based, the aims of this study were as follows:

1. To explore the nature of the beliefs, knowledge, views and ideas in relation to the area of postnatal anti-D administration of those midwives who practise within the midwifery model and believe in the normality of the birth process.

2. To determine whether analysis of this knowledge adds to the debate and/or supports the development of an alternative paradigm from that which currently exists in relation to routine postnatal anti-D administration.

Ultimately it was hoped that, if an alternative paradigm could be shown to exist, the study might lead to the elaboration of further research questions in this area.

Planning the research

It is acknowledged that quantitative, experimental research evidence is not the only form of knowledge acceptable to and useful in the practice of midwifery. Midwives may use tacit knowledge or intuitive judgement, they may develop knowledge through their own experience and that of the women they serve, and through the use of their senses (Siddiqui, 1994).

Because the medical model traditionally uses a positivist, quantitative approach, and this study aimed to explore other types of evidence, qualitative methods were considered the most appropriate. An inductive approach allows theory development through more subjective data, which embrace participants' philosophical beliefs rather than attempting to remove these from data analysis for fear of bias. Bates (1995) suggests that qualitative research is highly valid for midwifery, as it focuses on the woman as a whole and does not reduce her to parts.

The desire to explore midwifery knowledge also led to a qualitative approach to sample selection; randomly sampling midwives with this subject and objective would have been unlikely to give the type of data needed for the study. It would not progress the study of this topic to know what percentage of midwives have alternative beliefs regarding anti-D; rather, we need to explore what these are in depth with a view to clarifying midwifery philosophy and knowledge in this area.

Grounded theory was eventually chosen as the most appropriate research method for this study. This was developed by Glaser and

Strauss (1967) as a means for eliciting the shared meanings inherent in particular situations (Morse, 1992). It has been described as a 'theory development method "grounded" in actual research information' (Hill Bailey, 1997). This approach was selected as the most appropriate in terms of specific qualitative research methodology, mainly because of this deliberate focus on ongoing development of theory, where analysis occurs as data are collected until a point of saturation is reached.

The basic assumption of this theory is that we do not know all that there is to know (Norager Stern, 1985). It entails making constant comparisons between data collected, and systematically coding information in order to identify themes and generate categories of information. A theory is then built through use of inductive and deductive activity (Forchuk and Roberts, 1993).

A combination of purposive and convenience sampling was employed in the first stage of this study, and initially the participants were targeted in three ways:

1. Colleagues who had expressed an interest in the area were invited to respond.

2. Midwives were invited to participate via midwife discussion lists on the Internet.

3. A short article outlining the study topic and questions was published in *Midwifery Today* (Wickham, 1998), a journal which promotes the midwifery model, and midwives were invited to respond.

These methods also led to a degree of 'snowballing', where participants told other midwives about this research; this led to more responses.

In the first wave of this research, responses were received from 17 midwives; five were colleagues, six responded to information on Internet discussion lists, and two responded to the *Midwifery Today* article. The other four had been given information either by participants, or by colleagues who had seen the original request. Responses were received from midwives in the UK, USA, Australia, New Zealand, South America, Japan, Israel and Holland. The midwives who included personal details in their response had been practising for between 4 and 27 years. All but three worked, or had worked previously, in home birth or other out-of-hospital settings, and nine had worked with women who were offered, but chose not to receive, anti-D.

In the initial study, it was made clear to participants at all stages that responses were being sought only from midwives, and not from other childbirth professionals such as doulas or childbirth educators. Although these professionals have valuable knowledge in their own right, the aim here was to focus on the midwifery body of knowledge. However, since the completion of this study, the research carried out has expanded to include a number of other people who have responded to the ideas, presentations and articles on this topic. There has been the opportunity to expand the research in many ways and, while the material presented in this book remains in the format of the original study and responses, it has also been refined and expanded by subsequent work and research with other midwives, women and health experts. Having said this, it can still be argued that this fits into what is generally known as the midwifery model, as all of those who participated in the research are proponents and supporters of this model. The most recent estimate is that around 63 people from 13 countries have participated in this study in a significant manner.

In order to collect data in this area, midwives were initially asked to provide written responses detailing their beliefs, thoughts, feelings and experiences in this area. The rationale for utilizing written media (including electronic mail) was that it would be possible to embrace a global perspective and include midwives from different countries, systems of care and cultural backgrounds within this study, in order to gain as broad a picture as possible. Although this approach may be less efficient than interviewing in eliciting every nuance of meaning, it was felt justifiable in this case because of the advantages of the global perspective.

Having designed this original plan for data collection, it became apparent during the research that it was necessary to develop more of a dialogue with respondents, in order to clarify meaning and extrapolate the rich data that are a feature of this type of research. Therefore, semi-structured interviews and focus groups were conducted with participants. With those whom it was impossible to meet or speak to directly (usually because of geographical barriers), e-mail dialogue was used. Although this had been anticipated to be perhaps not the most effective method, it was actually as fruitful as interviewing, while less time-consuming.

After the original part of the research was completed, the data collection continued in this eclectic manner, with e-mail dialogue, personal dialogue, written material and group discussion being the most common forms used. The new or salient points from this later data were used to broaden the discussion in the following chapters.

The data were analysed on an ongoing basis. Responses were studied several times and broken down into initial categories emerging through the responses. As categories emerged, these were refined and linked according to the emerging data. As the data were read, transcribed and coded, a process of categorization emerged. A wide range of areas relating to this issue had been covered, although the overall themes seemed to be 'exploration' and 'explanation'. Several of the original categories were integrated in order to see the general themes that emerged and, as a result of this, some categories contained a larger amount of information, which was originally grouped into sub-categories.

Quotations used in the text are taken directly from original written responses and transcripts of original interview tapes. The only alterations made to written material were to correct spelling errors and to change American spellings to English versions for the sake of consistency. Additions needed for clarity have been placed in square brackets. Midwives in some countries refer to anti-D by the product name 'rhogam', and, as the terms are used interchangeably, this has not been altered.

Participants had used a wide variety of sources of knowledge to inform their responses, and some of the midwives who responded by mail or e-mail sent references, case studies or other material to support their statements. In some cases, the references had not previously been uncovered in this study (usually because the papers had been published overseas). Some of these data are included in the following chapters, along with other material sought following the initial analysis of results. The intention here is not necessarily to challenge or attempt to evaluate the views of the midwives, but to demonstrate where the findings are supported by other material.

An entire chapter on the research process is included for several reasons. First, it is sometimes frustrating to read texts that outline 'findings' without giving the reader the chance to assess the methodology or process of attaining those findings. I also wanted to emphasize the link between the nature of the data collection and the nature of the results of this study, because the eclectic, holistic and woman-centred way of collecting material led to similar kinds of data being offered. The other part of this rationale is that I wanted other midwives, who may not have been exposed to the research process in action, to see how such research was carried out, not least because demystifying this may make such research more accessible.

It is important to consider the reliability and validity of any research study. In general, efforts were made to ensure that participants' responses were used accurately and in context, and elements of a hermeneutic approach, where participants validate the findings of the study, were utilized once the results had been collated. During the final part of the initial study, it was possible to 'check back' with five of the original participants, who all agreed that the findings of the study accurately represented their original meaning. Two of these participants also commented that they felt the collation of the data they gave with that from other midwives had led to the development of a broad and useful theory in this area.

CHAPTER SIX

Philosophy and the question of iatrogenesis

No intervention is necessary on a routine basis.

In terms of their philosophy, most of the midwives who participated in this research felt that there was no such thing as an intervention which was justifiable on a routine basis. This was hardly surprising, considering that this research targeted midwives who 'trusted birth' and supported the midwifery model. Perhaps the most overwhelming feeling that came through the data was that midwives felt there had to be some sort of 'explanation' for the need for anti-D, and that this information was vital to women. Several of the midwives began their responses by saying or writing something like:

> I don't know if my experience can help you, but I would love to see what you find out; this is a really important issue.

> Your questions are important for all midwives to think about and use in the formulation of anti-D protocols in their care plans. The use/abuse of anti-D in {participant's country} is rife. We tend to over-use this very expensive resource.

This not only demonstrates the feelings of the midwives towards the subject area, but also confirms the relevance of this research question to midwifery practice. While this may not be the only routine intervention that remains unchallenged, it is certainly one of the few areas where it would be a struggle to find a view other than that espoused within the medical model.

Almost all of the participants directly stated that they felt that anti-

D was probably not necessary on a routine basis, and a number of reasons were given for this:

> I do not think rhogam is necessary on a routine basis because of the associated expense/maternal risk factors. I only arrange for the administration of anti-D to my clients if there is a clinical indicator for its use during pregnancy or after birth.

> {The} side effects of anti-D are so under-researched ... I find it so difficult to tell women that they need this, when I just don't know if that's true. Or to tell them that it's safe.

> I KNOW {participant's emphasis} in my heart that rhogam is not necessary for all of these women. All of my experience as a midwife confirms to me that birth works. I just wish I knew why ... {and} exactly what affected this.

> I just find it incredibly hard to accept that there is such a huge loophole in such a sophisticated system.

This 'midwifery model' perspective – that anti-D is not necessary on a routine basis, and that there is likely to be an explanation for the occasional transplacental haemorrhage in physiological birth – contrasts vividly with the stance of the medical model, where rhesus isoimmunization is seen to be akin to a potential disease requiring preventative treatment. Midwives who responded often explicitly stated that they felt there was not enough 'midwifery knowledge' in this area, and the differences between the medical and midwifery paradigms were clearly illustrated in the data collected.

The need for anti-D: historical factors

> If anti-D *is* necessary for some women, there must be a reason why.

One of the themes that emerged was the question of whether some women's need for anti-D had been caused by another factor. Again, this perspective contrasts with the medical view that the need for anti-D is inherent and a result of an immunological 'malfunction' or the existence of pathology in all rhesus-negative women's bodies. Some midwives felt that anti-D may be necessary for some women because of a form of 'unnatural intervention', although speculation in this area took two very different directions. It was clear from the data that midwives did not believe that pathology on this scale could be inherent in nature; instead, they offered explanations as to why isoimmunization might occur in a population that was otherwise well-equipped to nurture and give birth to babies.

The cause of isoimmunization?

It was suggested by some midwives that we might look to 'genetic intermingling' for an explanation of why anti-D has become necessary for some women:

> I always thought that originally the gene for rhesus negativity had been confined to one geographical area, maybe like sickle cell, although I'm not sure if it's quite the same. As we developed transportation, people from different areas mixed and had children. So rhesus-positive men from elsewhere began to have babies with rhesus-negative women and the problem began. I don't know if it's quite that simple, though.

This viewpoint suggests that women's bodies evolved without inherent pathology, but that the human race could have brought this pathology into the picture as a consequence of travel and racial and social interbreeding. This may explain the apparent aberration in the ability of some women's bodies to give birth to a series of healthy babies without intervention, and midwives have considered and offered evidence that suggests that various peoples and areas have historical and modern-day differences regarding the incidence of rhesus-negative women:

> Rh neg is very rare in Sioux and Assinaboine tribes.

> Being rhesus negative is unknown in Samoa.

> In Japan there are considerably fewer rhesus-negative women than in the West.

> Several thousand years ago, Rh– trait was confined to one specific Caucasian group, the modern-day Basques ... initially all other races were Rh+ve.

Whether or not this theory is true, the emergence of this theme again underlines the way that the midwifery paradigm does not accept that women are 'automatically defective', but rather seeks an explanation for the need for anti-D. In order to try to offer a discussion regarding this aspect of the results, a number of historians, anthropologists and other experts were approached. Unfortunately it has not been possible to find anyone who is able to offer an expert opinion in this complex and specific area (although any such comments would be gratefully received). Therefore, the following reflection has come from discussions with these academics and reading in related disciplines.

It goes without saying that, just as in midwifery, other academic disciplines generate schools of thought that are markedly different from each other. Egyptology is a classic example of a discipline with a school of traditional thought that is currently being challenged by a number of researchers who are looking at the evidence in new ways and proposing different theories. There are fundamental disagreements concerning the age of the Pyramids and the Sphinx and the nature of the societies who built them (Alford, 1998). This seemingly unrelated example may be relevant in illustrating one of the key points here; that if researchers who are experts in their own fields cannot agree on exactly how old the human race is, whether prehistoric societies were able to travel between continents, or what the origin of their superior technology might be, then it becomes incredibly difficult to extrapolate that evidence for use within another field. In the same way, we cannot comment specifically on the possibility that there was ever a time when people lived according to rhesus groups; for this is the starting point of such a theory.

The medicalization of birth

Along with the theory that anti-D is not necessary for all women came the suggestion that medicalization of the birth process may have increased the rate of rhesus sensitization:

> I know what the studies say about 13 per cent or something like that of women being sensitized anyway, and I wonder this ... we were doing managed third stage at that time, and all women got an epis{iotomy}. Well, I wonder how many of those women would have been sensitized if we had done more physiological third stages; whether that was causing higher rates of sensitization than might happen in a normal population of women who had natural birth.

This midwife is correct in pointing out that all of the clinical trials for anti-D were carried out after birth had become a medical event, and not before. This is one of the major problems with the research in the area; while we know that around 10 per cent of women who experience medical management of birth, and particularly the third stage of labour, will need anti-D to prevent isoimmunization, we do not know what percentage of women who experience physiological birth will need this. Again, the fundamental question here is whether transplacental haemorrhage is an occasional event in physiological birth, or whether this is frequent even without the addition of procedures that may cause it.

We do not even know which interventions women in the clinical trials experienced, even though this may have considerable impact on the results. When such a trial is conducted, we need to be sure that women in both the control and intervention group had similar experiences; for instance, it would be helpful to know whether the rate of induction of labour was the same in both groups of women. If it was higher in one group, then the results may be less valid. It is also helpful to know whether certain interventions correlate with a higher chance of transplacental haemorrhage. In the control groups of women who did not have anti-D, did more of the women whose labours were augmented develop antibodies than those whose labours were not augmented? These data would enable us to learn far more about this area; without it, we can only ponder the possibilities.

The suggestion that, at present, there may be 'no return' from the effects of this medicalization of birth was also discussed:

> We really don't know what the rate of sensitization is without medical intervention, and I bet we couldn't do research to find out now either.

It is certainly the case that it is far easier to introduce widely an intervention that is perceived to be useful than it is to remove that intervention, even when it has been shown to be useless or even harmful. Routine electronic fetal monitoring in labour is a classic example of this; while it is well documented that this serves not to improve outcomes but only to cause further intervention in labour, it remains a tool that is still widely used. In the case of anti-D, the issue is even more complex.

In order to carry out a randomized controlled trial to test whether electronic fetal monitoring is beneficial, women need only consent to having their baby monitored in different ways, such as with a pinard stethoscope or a hand-held doppler. Any trial that involved removing anti-D from women would entail those women taking the risk that they may become isoimmunized. Even if a proportion of women were happy to be part of such a study, perhaps because they had completed their family or were philosophically opposed to receiving anti-D, it seems extremely unlikely that such a study would attract the funding necessary to set it up and run it.

The other possibility is that of conducting research that looked at women who were declining anti-D anyway, and comparing their outcomes in relation to the kind of birth they experienced. However, would it be ethical, in the light of current knowledge, to suggest that a group of these women should experience any form of medical management unless this is genuinely essential for their wellbeing or that of their baby? The only truly ethical study may be one that looks at the outcomes of women who plan a physiological birth and are declining anti-D for their own reasons. In this area the concept of a randomized trial may not be compatible with the ethical issues involved, yet in reality many of us work in systems where decisions are made for women, and many of those making the decisions about women's care are biased towards the randomized controlled trial and away from other forms of evidence.

While the evidence that medical management may cause transplacental haemorrhage may be compelling for some, and even supported by some of the medical research (e.g. Katz, 1969), more work is needed in the area of physiological birth. Accepting that medical intervention may cause transplacental haemorrhage does not mean that we are in a position to give women an accurate estimate of the likelihood that they will experience this in a physiological birth. However, this is the one piece of evidence we desperately need to be able to give women. We know that the figure would be lower than 10 per cent; the question is, how much lower?

Following the discussion of iatrogenesis came the suggestion that the rate of isoimmunization in physiological birth may be so low that giving anti-D to all women would no longer be justified by a risk–benefit analysis:

> And if we knew what the real rate {of isoimmunization in physiological birth} was, well maybe the risks of anti-D would be a more relevant factor. We should be looking at the data for real

women – individually and now – not the population that had their birth messed with in 1969!

While women themselves may want to weigh up the risks and benefits of anti-D, those making decisions on a wider scale are often more interested in the cost-effectiveness of this product. Most of the debates concerning this have concluded that routine administration of postnatal anti-D is the most economic option. While there are certainly compelling arguments against basing decisions only on financial cost, these are perhaps less relevant here than the nature of the data used to inform such studies. The research examining the cost-effectiveness of anti-D (whether this is postnatal or antenatal) is based only on the data currently available. How much money could be saved if it was found that reducing certain unnecessary interventions reduced the need for anti-D? As noted in Chapter 3, around £1.3 million per year is spent in the UK on postnatal anti-D alone, a figure that might be massively reduced if we could determine which women really needed anti-D. Unfortunately, we only need to look at how much money is being made from the sale of anti-D, and we may have a clearer idea of whether this research is likely to be funded, supported or widely disseminated.

It was also suggested that the medical profession's philosophy of 'life at all costs', which the midwives concerned felt was characteristic of modern society, needs to be challenged in order to improve the long-term health of the population:

> I know this will be really controversial, but I don't think all babies were meant to live. And sometimes I think by making them live, we cause more problems than we solve. Or prevent.

> We don't all agree with fertility treatment, or keeping babies alive in neonatal intensive care units who have little chance of happy lives. We have to recognize that we might be doing the same thing by ignoring the implications of giving rhogam to all women. I mean, in terms of the gene pool.

> I think the medical profession has a lot to answer for, here and in other areas of practice. They are so keen to save, save, save. But do they think hard enough about the consequences, or alternative ways of doing it?

Again, the philosophical debate goes hand-in-hand with the clinical issues. Increasingly, midwives are questioning the effects of the roller coaster of medicalized birth on women and babies, and there is increasing evidence that the inappropriate use of technology and pharmacology leads to more problems than their proponents can hope to prevent.

There are many aspects to this debate; the first being the impact of scientific rationalism and the increasing number of new technologies on our culture. Many have noted that, for several decades, we have been progressing far faster in terms of our ability to achieve scientific goals than in our capacity to consider the implications:

> Do you remember that line in Jurassic Park, where the mathematician says to the scientists who've regenerated dinosaurs, 'You were so busy trying to find out if you could, that you didn't stop to think about whether you should.'

How true is this of the so-called advances in birth technology? We need only to think of relatively recent examples such as thalidomide or diethylstilboestrol, both of which were hailed as wonderful advances, only to be proven far more harmful than anyone had imagined. There may not be any actual evidence to suggest that anti-D is harmful on the same scale, yet how many people have really questioned the effect of anti-D programmes on the gene pool, or looked at the potential impact of this on growing babies?

There is little evidence in the literature that these theoretical and philosophical questions have been raised. Indeed, the product was developed and introduced within an incredibly short space of time as far as pharmaceutical products are concerned. While acknowledging that this was because it was genuinely believed that this was a wholly beneficial thing for women, the fact that these important questions remain must surely indicate that there is still work to be done in this area, certainly before mass programmes of antenatal administration are introduced. Whether or not we actually find potential problems upon analysis, surely we owe it to ourselves to ask these questions.

Finally, the point was made by midwives that rhesus disease may, if left alone, have been a relatively self-limiting condition. One midwife summarized this feeling by saying:

> Ironically, it may be because we have placed such a high value on the individual human life that, on a population level, we are going to suffer the consequences. I say ironically, because

doctors tend to ignore the individual in favour of the population in their research. It's a bit of a paradox when you think about it.

It certainly is ironic that, while the gold standard of medical research is the randomized controlled trial, which generally looks at the risks and benefits of an intervention on a population level, it is individual women who have to make the decisions – and individual women may not always find these kind of data helpful. Yet this midwife is suggesting that, in a system where individual lives are deemed so valuable, harm may be caused to society in general. This is another controversial issue, which we have perhaps not considered in as much depth as we could. What is the impact of this type of programme on the health of the population? Many medical advances that at one time appeared hugely advantageous are now being shown to cause problems. How can women be expected to make these decisions without being aware of the debates?

A number of midwives felt the need to 'follow the party line' on anti-D, whatever their personal beliefs and feelings about the product. One midwife encapsulated this theme when she explained that she cares both for 'country women', who have home births and do not even know their blood type, and for women in an urban area who, historically, have come to see obstetric intervention as the norm. Although she does not believe anti-D is necessary in physiological birth, and does not find that the 'country women' want this, she stated that:

> The truth is, I have gone along with this protocol {giving postnatal anti-D} mostly to continue to promote a sense of my midwifery being a responsible, professional type of midwifery, since this seems important as midwifery is not well recognized among the urban population quite yet.

How many midwives around the world are giving anti-D not because they feel it is a worthwhile or necessary intervention for women, but because they feel they must adhere to the medical model perspective and guidelines? And how does this impact on women? It would seem that the medicalization of birth has had an enormous impact on women and babies, and the anti-D programme is only one example of this. What recommendations would a consensus conference of women and midwives make in this area? Would they continue to give this product to all women, or work on finding out who would really benefit, and perhaps make greater efforts to remove unnecessary medical intervention from the birth process in order to reduce the impact of this on women's health and their need for further interventions?

CHAPTER SEVEN

Clinical and immunological factors

Another major theme of the research comprised a number of factors not previously cited in this debate and which participants thought were involved in isoimmunization. These data form the basis of this chapter and the two that follow. This chapter primarily considers the immunological and clinical factors that may mitigate the likelihood of isoimmunization in rhesus-negative women. Issues concerning the physiology of the placenta and the third stage of labour formed a major part of this theme; the data on these areas were so extensive that they have been considered as a separate issue in Chapter 8. Midwives also mentioned a number of lifestyle, nutritional and similar factors which were thought to impact on the likelihood of isoimmunization; these formed a further area of debate and reflection, which is discussed in Chapter 9.

The need for anti-D: factors limiting sensitization

Birth works; if you trust, understand and respect it.

In Chapter 6 it was noted that, in contrast with the medical view in this area, midwives generally felt that transplacental haemorrhage was not an inevitable part of pregnancy or birth. Yet rather than simply tabling this theory, the data they offered suggested that they had observed women and physiological birth to a degree that enabled them to identify factors from their experience which may well mitigate the chances of this event happening. As well as using personal reflective processes to consider such evidence, more than one midwife mentioned that she had discussed this aspect of her knowledge with other colleagues, sometimes in order to correlate what she had seen or surmised in relation to the experience of others.

Each of the factors cited has been considered in relation to the existing evidence in this area, and the data presented have been reflected upon and discussed with a number of experts in the relevant fields in order to allow comment on the suggestions. While there are as yet no quantitative studies that can help prove or disprove some of the evidence given here, readers may agree that extrapolation of evidence from other sources is a useful tool for reflecting upon the issues and judging whether further research may be beneficial.

Immunological factors

Midwives who addressed this area were often very specific about the factors they saw as limiting isoimmunization. The example below is representative of the kind of initial response received from midwives via e-mail or letter. Receiving this type of response confirmed the validity of requesting written replies to the questions – midwives were able to formulate sophisticated, detailed and technical information into logical and coherent structure, perhaps to a greater extent than they might have been able to do verbally:

My understanding is that the factors which LIMIT sensitization are:

1. ABO incompatibility (any fetal cells that gain entry into the maternal circulation are destroyed by maternal AB antibodies; there is a 90 per cent destruction with anti-A and a 55 per cent destruction with anti-B before any anti-D is formed)

2. Heterozygosity of the father. (If a recessive d gene is passed across during fertilization ... even though the father shows up as Rh +ve the baby will be Rh -ve)

3. Undetectable sensitization (sometimes so minimal it is not detected)

4. A natural immune defect (there is lack of antibody development to the Rh antigen, i.e. there is not a good complex between fetal and maternal cells).

ABO incompatibility

The issue of the 'natural' protection from isoimmunization conferred by ABO incompatibility was raised a number of times:

ABO incompatibility may confer a degree of protection against isoimmunization – antigens to A and B cells destroy fetal blood before production of anti-D occurs.

If a mother and her baby are ABO incompatible then I tend to assume that any fetal cells which do escape {into the maternal circulation} will be destroyed this way. But I would use this together with other factors anyway – I would still suggest a Kleihauer but I would be more assured that a Kleihauer which showed no fetal cells was correct in an ABO incompatible mom and baby than in an ABO compatible pair, where I might continue to look for clinical evidence.

Midwives were aware that this had been discussed in 'the research literature', although some stated that they were unsure whether medical colleagues accepted this as a valid reason to decline anti-D. ABO incompatibility is said to exist where a woman is blood group O and her unborn baby is blood group A, B or AB. Because people who are blood group O carry antigens to blood types A and B (and therefore AB), these antigens are able to destroy any of the baby's blood cells that may enter the maternal circulation before the woman's blood can produce antibodies to the rhesus antigen (Hoffbrand *et al.*, 1999).

Clarke *et al.* (1958) and Nevanlinna and Vainio (1956) both showed that ABO incompatibility between a woman and her baby offered protection against rhesus disease in the early years of anti-D research. However, research into the protection offered by ABO incompatibility did not continue, as it was thought to be 'unpromising'. Somewhere around 20 per cent of rhesus-negative women and their babies are ABO incompatible (Hoffbrand *et al.*, 1999), which means that up to one-fifth of all rhesus-negative women could potentially avoid the need for anti-D in this way. Yet the research that would establish the nature of this protection has not been carried out. It is a relatively simple matter to determine the baby's blood group, and this may be one of the key ways in which rhesus-negative women could be given more choice about this aspect of their pregnancies.

Other immunological factors
Four other immunological factors were discussed in relation to the likelihood of transplacental haemorrhage. The first of these concerned the 'Du' blood test result, which shows that a woman is weakly rhesus positive. Even though on some tests these women may appear to be rhesus negative, they are functionally the same as rhesus-positive women and therefore do not need to consider anti-D (Hoffbrand *et al.*, 1999).

Admittedly this is a small proportion of women, and some may not feel it is justified to attempt to use this evidence to inform practice. My responses to this would be twofold. First, if we put together all of the small groups of women, we might end up with a significant sized group of women who could be helped with further information concerning their need for anti-D. Secondly, we have already seen the implications of administering routine interventions on a population basis; surely the only way forward is to consider each woman individually and look at the factors that might make a particular intervention useful or otherwise for her?

It was also suggested that if a very small amount of fetal blood crosses over into the maternal circulation, there might be a natural mechanism for detecting and destroying these cells without producing anti-D. This is a very difficult proposition to prove or disprove; it impacts on the debate concerning sensibilization, which has already been discussed, and I suspect that only further work within a different philosophical model to that already used would enable light to be shed on this suggestion. It seems feasible that, although anti-D is generally produced in response to the entry of fetal blood into the maternal circulation, this may not be the only possible response to this event. Our understanding of possible explanations for the existence of such a phenomenon is limited only by our ability to step outside the current knowledge base in this area and consider other possibilities. Can we safely assume that we know all there is to know about the physiological mechanisms in an area that has been dominated by assumptions of pathology? The fact that this small study generated so many data which are contrary to some of the existing widespread assumptions would seem to support the suggestion that we should not continue to make such assumptions, but remain open to these other possibilities.

A 'natural immune defect' is thought to occur in some women, which prevents isoimmunization even if fetomaternal haemorrhage occurs. The term 'immune defect' is an interesting one to reflect upon in relation to current medical understanding in this area. It is assumed by the medical model that pregnant women are immuno-suppressed (a state in which their immune systems and ability to 'detect and deter' foreign matter function less well than normally) and that this is beneficial for their developing babies. Because the baby contains not only the genetic material from the mother but also that from the father, and because this material from the father could be recognized as foreign by the mother and consequently rejected, the physiological immunosuppression of pregnant women acts to prevent this occurrence.

Yet the theory of immunosuppression is only that – a theory. Again, perhaps we should consider the fundamental assumptions made in this area and reconsider the context in which these assumptions are based. Are all women truly immunosuppressed during pregnancy? How does this fit into a model of physiology? Could there be other possible explanations for this, and how would it impact on pregnant women? Is it also possible that the pathological type of immuno-suppression that may be seen in certain circumstances in the general population differs from a physiological immunosuppression that may occur during pregnancy? If this was the case, our understand-ing of this difference might have major implications within the area of rhesus sensitization. While we understand that the pregnant woman has a 'modified immune system', we know little about what the implications of this might be (Michel Odent, personal corre-spondence).

This discussion also relates to the final suggestion in this area. It was suggested that one of 'nature's reasons' for immuno-suppression in pregnancy was to ensure that women did not produce antibodies to fetal blood. This suggestion builds upon the theory that immunosuppression is a physiological aspect of preg-nancy, although it is not at odds with the idea that this immuno-suppression may not be pathological in nature. We therefore need to reflect upon two issues in this area; the evidence for immunosup-pression during pregnancy and the way this relates to isoimmuniza-tion within a physiological model, and the idea of a 'natural immune defect'. Clearly, in order to be able to reflect upon the latter, we may need to reconsider what we believe to be the 'truth' regard-ing the former.

Evidently there is more to be debated in terms of the physiology of the immune system and the process of isoimmunization itself; the work that has been carried out within the framework of the medical model is confined within the prerequisite assumptions held by that model. Yet this Western medical model is only one of many philosophies and modalities of healing; other philosophies concerning health will have different ideas about this. Certainly the concept that normal pregnancy is an immunological 'problem' is in conflict with the evidence which supports birth as a natural and social event. This alone begs many questions for future debate in this area.

Physiological and clinical factors

As already noted, midwives felt that isoimmunization was not a normal feature of normal birth, although several stressed that we may need to re-define what we mean by 'normal birth', because they felt we had moved far from this through the process of medicalization. A better term for our purposes might be 'physiological birth', which at least implies the absence of both pathology (whether actual or perceived) and intervention. Both trust in birth and the physiology of this process – particularly in relation to the third stage of labour, which forms the subject of Chapter 8 – were discussed by midwives:

> Isoimmunization doesn't worry me all that much. I know of several older women with negative blood types who had 13 children and never had rhogam. I tend to trust that nature knows what it does.

In order to support statements such as these, a number of physiological and clinical factors were cited by midwives as mitigating the likelihood of isoimmunization. Those presented here include a list of clinical and medical factors that midwives felt increased the likelihood of this. The most commonly cited clinical factor was the nature of the third stage of labour; because the data on this were so extensive, this has been considered separately.

Interventions in pregnancy, labour and birth were also thought to increase the possibility of fetomaternal transfusion. Most of those mentioned are features of medically managed birth. As well as those which are already known and discussed in this field (for instance, amniocentesis and external cephalic version), midwives also cited ultrasound scanning, exogenous oxytocin, intrauterine catheters, episiotomy, fundal pressure, directed pushing and the use of local and epidural anaesthetics (which include vasodilating drugs). Each of these has been considered below, together with the rationales given by the midwives for their inclusion and any existing evidence that may relate to this.

Ultrasound scanning

Ultrasonography was felt to be a risk factor for transplacental haemorrhage in two ways. The first concerns the potential trauma that may be caused to the placenta by the movement of the transducer over the abdomen. Midwives noted that a number of women have their placenta attached to the anterior wall of their uterus, which is where the transducer is moved during a scan. It was argued that the pressure applied to the transducer in order to visualize the relevant parts of the uterus, baby and placenta might in some cases cause a small part of the placenta to separate from the wall of the uterus, and thus cause bleeding from fetal vessels into the maternal circulation. It is possible that this is multi-factorial; for instance, this might only occur where the placental was not optimally healthy. It is known that babies tend to 'jump around' during ultrasound scans, perhaps to move away from the ultrasound itself (David, 1975; Lambley, 1985; Lawrence Beech and Robinson, 1996). It is not outside the bounds of possibility that this movement, which has been described by some expectant mothers as 'thrashing' (Lambley, 1985), may lead to a higher risk that the baby may cause slight damage to the cord or placenta.

The other question raised by midwives was the effect of the ultrasound waves themselves on the integrity of the placenta. As Lawrence Beech and Robinson (1996) highlight, very little is known about the effects of ultrasound on the baby, and even less concerning the implications for the placenta. Will we continue to fail to inform women about the lack of evidence concerning the safety of such procedures, or is it about time that women were enabled to make up their minds about whether they choose to have scans on the basis of the evidence available, rather than being assured that, as a societal convention, this must automatically be a good thing to do?

Exogenous oxytocin

The term 'exogenous oxytocin' describes the synthetic form of this otherwise naturally occurring hormone, which may be given to women in order to induce or augment their labour. (It is also used in relation to the third stage of labour, as discussed in Chapter 8.) Commonly used proprietary names for this drug include syntocinon (UK) and pitocin (USA). Usually administered in the form of an intravenous drip, exogenous oxytocin is becoming increasingly popular in hospitals, mainly because of a lack of understanding of birth physiology. Because this relates to several of the other suggestions here, these issues are discussed in depth.

It is well understood that when a labouring woman perceives danger her body will produce adrenaline (the 'fight or flight' hormone), which prepares her body to deal with the danger and also inhibits oxytocin. This can be explained as a helpful mechanism if we consider birth in the animal kingdom, where an animal that senses danger during labour will use this mechanism to stop her labour so that she and her family or pack can move to a place of safety. This response is clearly beneficial, allowing the animal to give birth only where she and her young will be safe. Exactly the same process occurs in humans, and can be seen where women leave home to go to a hospital with regular and strong uterine contractions, only to find that these stop or slow down upon arrival. While the rational part of her brain may have felt that the hospital was a 'good and safe' place to give birth, a more primitive part of her brain does not truly feel safe in this environment.

Sadly, many of those involved in hospital birth fail to understand this physiological process. While the logical response to this would be for attendants to ask whether the woman would prefer to return home, or to offer her and her partner a cosy room where they can be alone and wait for the onset of further contractions, this rarely happens in practice. It is far more likely that the cessation or decline of contractions will be seen as a sign of the woman's body 'failing to progress' (thereby neatly placing blame on the woman rather than the hospital or attendants), and that she will be given intravenous oxytocin.

The midwives in this study believed this to be a risk factor for transplacental haemorrhage because of its effect on the body. Where a woman produces her own oxytocin, this is carefully controlled by her body so that she only produces as much as she needs at any given time. She might produce more towards the end of the first stage of labour, as the last part of her cervix is drawn up around her baby's head. Later, she may produce less as the cervix becomes fully dilated, in order to give her body a rest and enable the uterus to adjust its shape in preparation for the birth itself. Where exogenous oxytocin is administered, the quantity is controlled by the attendant and the volume infused usually only rises; thus the woman may be receiving more oxytocin than her body would have produced itself. It is this aspect which the midwives felt to be a danger, in that an overdose of oxytocin could lead to a degree of hyperstimulation of the uterus and extremely strong contractions, which could potentially cause the placenta to separate too early. This hyperstimulation may not always be detectable by attendants, especially those who are unused to assessing the progress of physiological birth.

The other problem caused by exogenous oxytocin is that it inhibits the woman's body's production of its own – endogenous – oxytocin (Robertson, 1997). Oxytocin is intimately involved in the separation of the placenta during the third stage of labour, which is the point felt by the midwives to be the most crucial in terms of transplacental haemorrhage. It seems logical that interference with the woman's production and regulation of this substance might indeed be a factor that affects her chance of experiencing a fetomaternal bleed and subsequent isoimmunization.

Intrauterine catheters

Some midwives suggested that these devices, which may be placed in the uterus of some women in order to monitor the strength of contractions, posed a potential danger to the integrity of the placenta. It is logical that any instrument inserted into the uterus, even with extreme care, may cause slight trauma to the placenta; slight trauma may be all that is needed for fetomaternal bleeding to occur during birth. Midwives also suggested that this kind of invasive medical intervention in labour generally could have an impact on the delicate hormonal balance that is needed for this to occur; such a suggestion supports the proposal that isoimmunization may be an iatrogenic consequence of the medical approach to birth.

Episiotomy

Episiotomy is also thought to be a risk factor for transplacental haemorrhage, as this is known to decrease the level of circulating endogenous oxytocin. As the baby's head distends the perineum, a neural message from the stretch receptors in this area causes a surge of oxytocin, which facilitates the physiological birth of the placenta and membranes. This process is timed with incredible precision, and the amount of oxytocin released is exactly that which is needed for the subsequent contractions in order to optimize the process of placental separation.

Episiotomy interferes with this process in that the cutting of the perineum results in the loss of the 'stretching message' that causes the oxytocin to be released, and thus a woman who has an episiotomy lacks the surge of oxytocin which facilitates the third stage (Robertson, 1997). This then means that placental separation is not optimal and, because it is the process of separation that is felt to be so crucial to the prevention of isoimmunization, this consequence is rendered more likely.

Fundal pressure

Fundal pressure may occur either deliberately, where attendants push on the fundus to attempt to expedite the birth of a baby or the placenta, or accidentally, where the woman is asked to adopt a position which puts unnecessary pressure on the top of her uterus. Again, midwives suggested that this could interfere with placental attachment and physiology, and potentially cause fetomaternal transfusion. Although there is a great deal of research suggesting that this is not beneficial in general, anecdotal evidence from midwives working in some hospitals would suggest that this is still employed by some practitioners. A variation of this is used in the medical management of the third stage (see Chapter 8).

Directed pushing

As with the addition of synthetic oxytocin to physiological birth, directed pushing (where an attendant instructs the woman when and how to push, rather than encouraging her to push instinctively and in response to her body's cues) was seen to be a potential cause of fetomaternal transfusion. Here, non-physiological pushing is thought to lead to increased intrauterine pressure, which may in turn cause trauma to the placental site or possibly the rupture of small vessels. Directed pushing usually involves the Valsalva manoeuvre, where the woman is instructed to take a deep breath and push for as long as she can. The fact that the Valsalva manoeuvre was originally invented as a method for forcibly removing pus from the ear would support the idea that this could create enough force to cause trauma elsewhere in the body. The Valsalva manoeuvre also causes changes in blood pressure and the amounts of oxygen and carbon dioxide in the woman's and baby's bloodstream; again, this may have an impact on placental circulation.

Local and epidural anaesthesia

The main concern with the use of epidural anaesthesia and local anaesthetics (such as those which might be used in preparation for episiotomy) is that the preparations used for these interventions often contain vasodilators; chemical substances that cause blood vessels to widen. These vasodilators may be carried through the body, potentially causing the dilatation of vessels in and around the placenta. Dilatation of these vessels may then lead to the escape of blood from fetal vessels, especially if this occurred around the time of the third stage. It is the practice of some practitioners to infiltrate the perineum with local anaesthetic and even to begin suturing tears or episiotomies before the placenta has delivered; this practice may also cause vasodilatation and inhibit the normal separation of the placenta.

Epidural anaesthesia was also seen as a potential problem for other reasons; this may lead to a number of other interventions, including the administration of exogenous oxytocin, instrumental delivery or Caesarean section, which themselves may increase the likelihood of transplacental haemorrhage. It was suggested that women wishing to avoid transplacental haemorrhage might choose to use non-pharmacological pain relief rather than pharmacological drugs.

The midwifery evidence that concerns specific interventions and the suggestion that these might interfere with normal physiology and cause fetomaternal transfusion can be neatly summarized in the words of the midwife participants:

> We must understand that everything, absolutely everything we do has implications for women and that we should consider any intervention in light of this. Even checking a woman {vaginally} might cause interference to a low-lying placenta.

> We need to respect birth and not mess with it unless we really have to. That's how it goes wrong, when we start to interfere with the normal and try and control things. We don't – well we can't – control it. Women's bodies and whatever force governs the universe does that. The sooner we can all learn that one, the better for everybody.

Other factors

The midwives' list of factors that might cause transplacental haemorrhage was not limited to those specifically linked with pregnancy and birth. It was also suggested that the question of why some women become sensitized is linked to environmental factors; examples given included fluoride, xenoestrogens, and other pollutants which may interfere with normal physiology and/or compromise a woman's immune status. The idea that these substances may lead to an increased likelihood of transplacental haemorrhage was immediately followed by the suggestion that pregnant and birthing women should minimize their exposure to these substances. These suggestions, and the evidence that may support or refute them, are considered in Chapter 9, along with data on natural substances and 'positive intercessions' which may actively help to prevent transplacental haemorrhage.

Implications of this evidence

The expansion of knowledge and understanding in this area means that we might have more information that would help us to identify which women may become isoimmunized, either during pregnancy or birth. This evidence may relate to the issue of antenatal anti-D; if more factors than originally thought might cause isoimmunization, then could this explain some of the instances of so-called 'silent' fetomaternal transfusion? Perhaps these events aren't all so silent after all. While there remains a need to discover to what extent each of these interventions might be involved in transplacental haemorrhage, this information might be beneficial to women who wish to avoid anti-D and who want to maximize their chances of avoiding fetomaternal haemorrhage. If some or all of these interventions (and, of course, there may be others to add to the list) were shown to cause this in a proportion of women, then individual women would be able to decide whether they wanted to have these interventions in the light of this evidence. If an individual woman felt an intervention to be justified, then she may want to consider antenatal anti-D at the appropriate time in her pregnancy.

It is acknowledged that, at present, few women are lucky enough to have the kind of physiological birth that is facilitated by the midwives who took part in this study. This is not because their bodies are not capable of undertaking this, but because they live in a culture that places a higher value on medicine and technology. While some might see this as confirmation that those women who give birth in hospital need routine anti-D, there are other, perhaps more positive, ways to interpret this information.

Some might feel that this evidence acts as further confirmation that medicalized birth is not necessarily the best option for the majority of women, and that intervention leads to further intervention. Certainly these data might help those women who wish to avoid anti-D; they would be well advised to consider giving birth in an environment which is conducive to physiological birth, such as at home or in a birth centre with midwives. They may also choose to avoid the interventions in pregnancy and labour that could increase the likelihood of transplacental haemorrhage. Even women who do not plan to give birth at home and are happy to have anti-D post-natally might wish to avoid interventions in pregnancy which may increase their likelihood of isoimmunization. The unknown risks of anti-D to an unborn baby cause more concern to some women than the potential risks to their own health.

Those midwives and other attendants who work with birthing women may find some value in the midwives' suggestion that interventions other than those currently understood to cause antenatal transplacental haemorrhage may occasionally lead to this. There is clearly a danger that proponents of routine anti-D will see the expanded list of interventions that could cause fetomaternal transfusion as a justification for the routine administration of this. There are two ways of looking at this information. One would be to say that, because most women have ultrasound scans, then they had better have antenatal anti-D as well. Yet a large number of women have scans in pregnancy, and they obviously do not all become isoimmunized as a result. We might surmise from this that there is not an automatic and direct correlation between the two, but rather that those women who experience medical interventions are at increased risk of transplacental haemorrhage.

The other way of using this information would then be to consider the issues further, with a view to informing women that they may be more likely to need anti-D if they choose to have other interventions in pregnancy and birth. Already there is plenty of information concerning the risks of such interventions, which women may or may not be offered by health professionals. Perhaps the addition of even more risks to the knowledge base surrounding these practices would lead to more attendants offering women accurate information upon which they can base their choices?

Above all, the message from the midwives seems to be that physiological birth is superior – both for women and babies – to a birth which is medically managed. This is not a new message, but neither is it one that is being heeded. Why do more woman not have the option of experiencing this kind of birth? It would seem from the evidence that there are several good arguments for the suggestion that medical management of pregnancy and birth may increase the occurrence of isoimmunization. While we certainly need to work on increasing the evidence in this area, we might simultaneously consider the issue of how physiological birth can become an option for all women.

CHAPTER EIGHT

Placental physiology and the third stage

In Chapter 7, a number of physiological and clinical factors which midwives suggested mitigated the likelihood of isoimmunization were discussed. Overwhelmingly, the clinical factor most commonly mentioned by the midwives was the third stage of labour. The data collected suggested that the development, physiology, separation and birth of the placenta were critical in this debate. This chapter considers the evidence in this area, both from the midwives in this study and from other sources. In order to present the issues within the context of placental physiology and the physiology of the third stage, these processes are outlined before the evidence from the midwives is presented.

Placental development and physiology

The placenta is a complex and intricate organ which is designed to act as a 'buffer' between maternal and fetal circulations, allowing oxygen, carbon dioxide, nutrients and waste substances to pass between the two without the mixing of blood itself. This is achieved by the development of villi, tree-like protrusions formed in the placenta which sit next to the maternal vessels, allowing the substances to cross via specialized cells and membranes. The placenta embeds in the uterine wall at the point of conception and grows with the baby to form the baby's 'lifeline'. The placenta plays an incredible role in the growth of a baby, and remains *in situ* until after the baby is born, when it then separates from the uterine wall and is itself 'birthed' during what has become known as the 'third stage of labour'.

Inch (1982) offers an extensive description of the physiology of the third stage, which is paraphrased in the following account. Once the baby is born, the uterus reduces in size and the placental site is also made smaller. This causes the placenta to be squeezed, and some of the maternal blood in the placenta moves into the uterine veins, causing the uterus to become tense. (The uterine muscles also play a part in retaining this tension.) At the same time, some of the fetal blood in the placenta is passed to the baby, enabling the placental wall to thicken further in preparation for separation.

As uterine contractions recommence, a few of the congested maternal vessels burst and the small amount of blood which is released causes the placenta to become detached from the uterine wall. This maternal blood causes the spongy lining of the placenta to separate from the uterine wall, and the 'living ligature' effect of the uterine fibres seals the maternal vessels and begins the process of healing. The blood that is lost is maternal; midwives will confirm from experience that the newly born placenta does not bleed from the attachment site. Even where a retroplacental clot has formed, this is as a result of maternal blood becoming congested on the surface of the placenta rather than an indication of the presence of fetal or placental blood.

It can be seen from the above that the placenta is intricately designed to ensure that the blood from the baby does not mix with that of the mother. Crucially, the blood that enters the uterus is maternal; the release of fetal blood does not play a part in the normal physiology of the third stage. Perhaps as a consequence of their knowledge in this area, the midwives in this study found it difficult to reconcile this remarkable feature of physiology with the idea that this anatomical and physiological design regularly fails during pregnancy and birth:

> Why is there a chorion and an amnion? We need to ask – why does the chorionic plate exist at all? Unless maternal and fetal circulations were not meant to mix.

> My belief is that transplacental haemorrhage does not occur during natural birth, as the layer of Nitabusch is designed to prevent this. If this layer of the decidua is healthy and not interfered with or traumatized during the birth process, no transfer of fetal cells into the maternal circulation will occur.

The placenta is an incredible organ ... It doesn't just fail, I don't believe that. It might be caused to fail by our interfering, but it doesn't fail just like that. Not more than a tiny percentage of the time, anyway, and we're not talking about a tiny percentage here, we're talking about a lot of alleged placenta failure!

The midwives suggested that the physiology of the placenta protected women from fetomaternal haemorrhage, again reiterating their belief that this was not a normal occurrence in physiological birth. They question the fundamental assumption made within the medical model perspective in this area: that transplacental haemorrhage is a common feature experienced by women during this time, again rendering pregnancy and birth inherently pathological.

The third stage of labour

The third stage of labour was seen as the most important aspect in this debate – perhaps because this is the time where the most potential for interference in placental physiology exists. As far as the midwives were concerned, the optimal third stage needs to occur physiologically without any attempt at 'management':

And when I say 'hands off', I mean that nothing at all should be done to the cord or the uterus or the placenta. We don't need to be fiddling, we need to be more patient and wait for things to happen. No touching the cord to see if it's pulsating – we'll know it's stopped when the placenta comes out. And I think even if we keep handling the uterus to see what we can feel we may be interfering with the normal separation. We need to trust more.

Oxytocic drugs and any degree of cord traction are thought to interfere with normal placental separation and render fetomaternal transfusion more likely. Touching or massaging the uterus unnecessarily at any stage may cause further bleeding and increase the chance of transplacental haemorrhage. Some aspects of this evidence were discussed in the previous chapter; this is supported by Katz (1969), who showed that trauma to the interior of the uterus increased the likelihood of transplacental haemorrhage.

A number of specific aspects of a managed third stage were expressly mentioned by the midwives as the interventions which they saw as being likely to cause fetomaternal haemorrhage. The first of these was the administration of an oxytocic drug, such as syntometrine or pitocin. It was felt that, because the action of this drug is to cause a massive contraction of the uterus, the contraction would cause the placenta to separate much faster and with more force than in a physiological separation. This may not allow time for the blood to transfer and the living ligature effect to take place, and may somehow enable fetal blood to enter maternal vessels. This may also cause the placental vessels to burst, which would not be a normal occurrence during this time.

The use of controlled cord traction was also seen as potentially harmful; again, the effect of an attendant pulling on the cord may be to cause parts or all of the placenta to separate before this would have occurred physiologically, with the same result. The pressure of an attendant's hand on the uterus, a procedure routinely used with controlled cord traction to 'guard' the uterus from being inverted, may also affect the delicate physiology of placental separation or cause fetal vessels to burst, in the same way that fundal pressure may lead to fetomaternal transfusion. Even touching the cord, perhaps to see if it is still pulsating, may potentially interfere with the balance of circulation between mother and baby. Finally, women experiencing managed third stage may be directed to push by attendants. Directed pushing may also cause unnatural pressure to build in the uterus, which may in turn cause vessels to burst or blood to be forced into the maternal circulation, and thus also be a risk factor for transplacental haemorrhage.

The physiology of the third stage itself also offers clues to confirm the protective nature of this process. Not only does the physiological mechanism prevent fetal blood from being released from the placental site, but the maternal blood may also act as a cleansing mechanism to prevent transplacental haemorrhage. Any fetal blood which had seeped from the placenta may be washed away (through the cervix and vagina) by the maternal blood, thus adding a further protective mechanism against transplacental haemorrhage. The only time when this mechanism might not be able to protect women is if they experienced a deep tear or episiotomy. It is then theoretically possible that, if something had interfered with the normal physiology of the third stage, any fetal blood that had been released might enter these vessels. Perhaps this would partially explain why, historically, traditional midwives so valued their skills in preventing perineal tears.

Guidelines for a physiological third stage

As well as giving details of those interventions that they felt should be avoided, midwives discussed the positive aspects of a physiological third stage which they felt were relevant in preserving placental physiology. These are presented below.

- The most frequently mentioned aspect was that the midwife (or other birth attendant) needs to enable the third stage to be physiological and ensure she doesn't interfere at all. This means that she must not touch any part of the woman, baby or cord unless this is vital. The only 'vital' time to touch a woman or the cord, for one midwife, was if the woman was bleeding heavily and in danger of becoming compromised by this.

- Midwives should also have a good working knowledge of the physiology of the third stage and related clinical issues, such as the signs of physiological separation of the placenta; it was also suggested that midwives should reflect on their experiences in order to develop knowledge for the future.

- As the baby is born, help the mother to 'catch' and hold the baby in any position that is comfortable for both. Help the woman to dry her baby and enable her to hold the baby against her skin; offer a warm towel or blanket to cover the baby. Do not separate the baby from the mother or otherwise touch the baby.

- Do not touch, cut or otherwise interfere with the cord. The only point at which the midwife needs to touch the cord or placenta is when the placenta is being born; she can then hold a receptacle underneath or gently 'catch' the placenta. Even at the stage, it is not helpful to pull the cord or placenta; very occasionally, a part of the placenta may still be attached to part of the uterus even when it is visible in the vagina.

- Do not touch the uterus unless to feel for a contraction; even in this case, it was suggested that experienced midwives have learned to keep their hands off the uterus and trust the woman to tell them when they experience a contraction. Uterine massage before placental separation can disturb the pattern of contractions and normal separation, lead to bruising and haematoma (El Halta, 1998), and increase the likelihood of transplacental haemorrhage.

- Enable the woman to adopt any position she chooses; most women, including those who have given birth in an upright position, will instinctively lie down for the third stage.

- Ensure the room is heated – it needs to be hotter for the third stage than for the birth itself. One midwife commented that if the midwife is not uncomfortably warm, then the room is not hot enough! This proposition is reiterated by Odent (1998) as important in facilitating the physiology of the third stage.

- Create an atmosphere of unhurried calm.

- Do not encourage or direct the woman to push; if she asks when to push, tell her to push when and how her body tells her to. Reassure her that it is normal not to feel a need to push for a while after the baby is born.

- Remember that a long third stage may not be pathological; unless the woman is bleeding heavily, there is no reason to hurry it. Women who have short labours may have longer third stages than normal. One midwife commented that the longest third stage she had ever seen lasted for several hours; upon delivery of the placenta the cord was found to have partially detached from the remainder of the placenta. Clearly, if this third stage had been hurried, or if anyone had pulled on the cord, the results could have been catastrophic.

The third stage debate

The way in which the third stage is conducted has been a topic of great debate among midwives recently. Having established that the midwives in this study feel that enabling women to have a physiological third stage is one of the keys to avoiding isoimmunization, it seems appropriate to look at the evidence concerning third stage. Is a physiological third stage a safe option for the majority of women?

The third stage debate essentially concerns the comparison of physiological third stage and 'managed' third stage. Generally, any form of interference in the third stage constitutes management. Even if an oxytocic is not given and controlled cord traction is not used, a third stage where the cord is frequently checked for pulsation, or where the mother is encouraged to push in order to deliver the placenta within a specified time limit, would not be considered physiological by those experienced in this.

Historically, the concern regarding physiological third stage has been that this leads to more blood loss than managed third stage; this has certainly been the main focus of the research trials that have been carried out in this area. The first of these is generally known as the Bristol Trial (Prendeville *et al*., 1988), and compared the outcomes of the third stages of 1695 woman who were randomized into two groups; those experiencing active management of their third stage and those experiencing physiological 'management'.

There were a large number of sources of potential bias in this trial, some of which may have seriously affected the outcomes. The design of the trial was changed part-way through; the criteria for entry into the trial was amended to exclude more women and to allow clinicians actively to manage the third stages of women in the physiological group if they deemed this necessary. Yet the data on those women who were switched to active management were still included in the physiological group. There is evidence that the outcomes of women experiencing physiological third stage improved as the study went on, suggesting that the experience of the attendant was an important feature of the outcomes of this.

Many of the women in the physiological group did not experience truly physiological third stage; for instance, over half of the women in this group had their cords clamped and cut before the placenta was delivered. This may be because the training that attendants received in physiological third stage was poor. Clearly, there was an existing bias towards active management and, as the trial could not be blinded or double-blinded, the perceptions of the clinicians regarding the style of management may have led to differences in their recording data, such as estimated blood loss.

In response to the perceived shortcomings of the Bristol Trial, a further trial was conducted in Hinchingbrooke 10 years later (Rogers *et al*., 1998). Unfortunately, this trial had some of the same problems; the definitions of physiological (or expectant) 'management' still included the possibility of cutting the cord before the placenta was born, and placed a 1-hour time limit on the delivery of the placenta, even in the absence of problems. The researchers failed to exclude from the study women experiencing one or more of a number of interventions that are known to pose an additional risk of postpartum haemorrhage, such as episiotomy and the use of systemic opiates (e.g. pethidine). Conceivably, this could have caused the rate of postpartum haemorrhage in the physiological group to rise artificially as a result. Because this study took place in a hospital where women experienced medically managed labours and births, this may also have impacted on the results. The sources of potential bias are enough to throw serious doubt on the validity or usefulness of the results.

There are several fundamental questions regarding the third stage that render such trials less than useful; the first concerns the definitions of postpartum haemorrhage. While the trials used absolute definitions of this in terms of the amount of blood lost (a postpartum haemorrhage was considered to be a blood loss of greater than 500 ml), experienced clinicians know that the amount of blood lost during the third stage does not always correlate with the physical symptoms of postpartum haemorrhage. Most experienced birth attendants will have observed women who have lost more than 500 ml of blood, yet suffer no ill-effects of this; it is also possible that women can lose less blood than this but, perhaps because of other factors, suffer as a result. It is such an individual situation that it is almost impossible to apply general outcome measures with any degree of accuracy.

In terms of philosophy, the medical model perspective on the third stage is that 'less loss is better'. However, this is not the case within other models of health, such as Chinese medicine. Holistic birth attendants are more open to the idea that, because blood volume increases in pregnancy, some women need to lose more blood during the third stage than others, yet will not suffer as a result. As Begley (1998) notes, 500 ml is roughly equivalent to the amount of blood 'lost' during routine blood donation, and blood donors are given tea and biscuits rather than intravenous transfusions. Why is this situation handled so differently when a woman has just given birth? This seems even more incongruous when we consider that women's blood volumes increase during pregnancy to help them cope with this loss at birth.

The evidence from holistic midwives who support and are experienced in physiological third stage would seem to bear out the suggestion that this does not cause greater blood loss than managed third stage, except in the hands of those who are not proficient at facilitating physiological processes. It is also possible that, even if the initial blood loss is lower with the use of oxytocic drugs, some of the blood that would have been lost may pool in the artificially contracted uterus and be released later. It is unlikely that this would be recorded in the woman's notes (Wickham, 1999c).

Perhaps the most pressing need in terms of research is to explore women's feelings about the third stage. Women's concerns have been neglected in the research trials carried out, and this would seem to be of vital importance to the debate. One aspect highlighted by the midwives in this study concerns the way in which some practitioners present managed third stage to women as a 'better option' because this takes less time. However, they may not tell women that they have a higher chance of needing to have their placenta removed under anaesthetic if they choose to have a managed third stage, a procedure which certainly does not save time. One of the midwives later commented that modern society seems to be preoccupied with speed, and questioned whether this attitude was detrimental in relation to birth. Certainly many of the interventions routinely introduced are seen by some to be superior to nature because they speed up the birth process, but it should be remembered that birth, women and babies often do not benefit from artificial acceleration.

There is general agreement amongst midwives and researchers that we have a need to explore the physiology of birth in far greater depth, with a focus on considering 'the normal'. This may be the single most relevant direction in which this research has pushed the boundaries of knowledge in this area. Odent (1998) discusses a similar issue, in surmising that we always talk about 'management' of the third stage, and consider physiological third stage to be characterized by the removal of interventions carried out in a 'managed' third stage, rather than positive intercessions. This may also be true in relation to rhesus sensitization; it may not only be about removing medical intervention from pregnancy and birth for those women who wish to avoid anti-D, but also about considering ways of maximizing their body's ability to undertake the complex physiological processes required. This concept is discussed further in Chapter 9.

Clamping the cord

The other area of the third stage that was discussed at length by midwives was the clamping of the umbilical cord; it was felt that this would interfere with normal physiology and potentially lead to transplacental haemorrhage. Gaskin had already raised this issue in 1989:

> Late cutting of the umbilical cord may also prevent a certain number of these blood sensitizations; when the cord is cut

before it stops pulsating, fetal blood may be forced backward from the placenta into the maternal circulation.

The midwives in this study noted that:

> Early cord clamping {before the birth of the placenta} can probably cause a fetomaternal bleed on its own ... It interferes with the circulations of mother and baby. Then the amount and circulation of blood in the placenta is going to be changed, so how can we expect the placenta to separate normally after that?

The idea that the cord is best left unclamped is supported by the work of Morley (1998), who began researching the idea of saving placental blood for transfusion into sick babies. He then found what he describes as a 'disturbingly obvious alternative', and showed that, 'if cord clamping is delayed to permit normal placental transfusion, the need for newborn transfusion could often be eliminated' (Morley, 1998). His work is supported by that of others, including Maisels (1992), who showed that leaving cords unclamped reduced blood loss and often the time taken for physiological third stage to occur. How long will proponents of the medical model take to realize that this kind of evidence, which often comes from obstetricians and paediatricians as well as midwives, may be more useful than trials which do not usefully tell us anything about third stage?

Indications of transplacental haemorrhage

One of the key issues in the anti-D debate concerns the nature of the Kleihauer test, and the fact that the inaccuracy of this makes it difficult to identify whether a woman has experienced transplacental haemorrhage. The widespread introduction of a more accurate test would be one of the keys to enabling informed choice in relation to the administration of anti-D. Yet the midwives in this study tabled the idea that we might not be reliant only on the use of such a laboratory test, in their suggestion that there are a number of clinical indications for transplacental haemorrhage:

> I believe that many women become sensitized because of an unnatural escape of fetal cells into their circulation e.g. during a Matthews–Duncan mechanism of placental separation, an extremely large placental site, or unnatural trauma at the site of implantation of the placenta, either during operative delivery or 'active management' of the third stage of labour.

Four indicators for determining whether transplacental haemorrhage had occurred were offered by midwives. This information applies to women who have otherwise experienced physiological birth and third stage, and therefore doesn't include those with medical interventions that midwives felt might cause transplacental haemorrhage.

1. *Matthews–Duncan separation may indicate transplacental haemorrhage.* While the placenta is normally born 'inside-out', in the amniotic sac, occasionally the placenta begins to separate from the uterus on one side, rather than in the middle. This is termed a 'Matthews–Duncan' separation, where the maternal side appears first and is followed by the membranes. While this is generally considered a normal alternative by midwives, it was suggested that this form of placental birth might indicate that separation of the placenta had not been completely normal; perhaps because more maternal blood tends to escape during this kind of separation. The midwives who cited this as an example of a situation where they might consider the risk of transplacental haemorrhage to be higher said they felt this information to be helpful where a woman was unsure about having anti-D and wanted to look at the evidence 'for and against' her having experienced transplacental haemorrhage.

2. *A particularly large placental site may indicate transplacental haemorrhage.* Again, a woman who had an especially large placenta was thought to be at higher risk of experiencing transplacental haemorrhage than a woman with an average-sized placenta. This may be because the larger placenta cannot be reduced in size as well as a more moderately sized placenta, causing some delay in the separation process or damage to fetal vessels on the placenta itself. It then follows that a woman giving birth to twins might also be more likely to experience fetomaternal transfusion.

3. *An abnormal pattern of bleeding during the third stage may indicate transplacental haemorrhage.* Clearly, in order to define an 'abnormal bleeding pattern' we need to consider what midwives see as normal bleeding during a physiological third stage. This is an issue that needs debate amongst those midwives who are experienced in physiological birth and third stage. While there is some evidence in this area, and a number of holistic midwives who possess this kind of knowledge, I am reluctant at this stage

to use the data to attempt to define the limits of normal third stage bleeding. It would seem more appropriate for this to be the subject of future research. One of the reasons for this is that the midwives in the original study emphasized that it would not be helpful to have a rigid or set pattern of normal blood loss, because this differed so much between women, but that, with experience, a midwife would be able to identify an unexpected pattern of bleeding at this time.

4. *Women may sense whether or not they have experienced transplacental haemorrhage.* While this is the suggestion that probably contrasts most strongly with the medical model beliefs about birth, a number of midwives told stories of midwives and women who had used intuition to inform their choices about anti-D. A few of these concerned women who had used meditation or intuitive processes to determine whether they felt they had experienced transplacental haemorrhage. Those open to the spiritual aspects of birth may more readily accept this as a valid tool for some women and midwives. For those who are more sceptical, the following explanation was given by one of the midwives who raised this as a possibility:

The starting point is to consider whether you accept that somewhere in the woman's body is the knowledge of whether some of the baby's blood has got into her blood. Somewhere, maybe in her blood, her body 'knows' that she has experienced this (or not). I obviously don't mean 'know' in the rational, brain-related sense of the word ... but her blood has to 'know' at some point, because if this knowledge wasn't there then antibodies wouldn't be formed.

So if we accept that this knowledge exists somewhere, then it is a shorter leap to accepting that this knowledge could be transferred from one area of her body to another ... from a kind of subconscious knowledge to a conscious knowledge. It's a lot shorter leap than asking someone to believe that you have knowledge of future events; you're only asking them to believe that people can have knowledge of what is happening in their own body ... at a time when they are particularly open to that knowledge.

A study on midwives' use of intuition was conducted by Davis-Floyd and Davis (1996), who gave numerous examples of midwives and women who had successfully used intuitive knowledge and processes to help inform their decision-making. There is little doubt that a fair proportion of midwives and women find intuition helpful in their lives. The really pertinent question becomes that which asks why intuitive knowledge has become so devalued in modern society in general, and in particular by proponents of systems of thought such as the Western medical model. For years it has been understood that many clinicians fail to listen and respond to women's needs, requests, knowledge or emotions (Graham and Oakley, 1991). Could this source of potential knowledge and insight add to the inevitably limited evidence that can be found through research? How can we enable women and their attendants to focus on this knowledge and consider its value in practice?

Yet again, the evidence presented highlights a contrast between the medical and midwifery models. Traditionally, work has focused on the assumption that transplacental haemorrhage is an undetectable and integral feature of birth, a theory that is compounded within the medical model by the inability of medical science to determine absolutely by laboratory testing whether this has occurred. The midwives here are suggesting not only that they believe fetomaternal transfusion is not inevitable, but that it may be predictable by clinical and other means. While the focus of the medical model is to 'seek problems', the midwifery model 'assumes normality until proven otherwise'.

Whether or not physiological third stage is the 'key' to the question of transplacental haemorrhage is a question that can only be answered for sure by further research. To date, all of the research into anti-D has been carried out on women who experienced hospital birth and managed third stage. Yet two things are certain: first, we have relatively little knowledge about the normal physiology of the placenta and the third stage of labour; and secondly, midwives who are open to the kind of thinking which expands their knowledge have a completely different perspective to that currently presented in the medical model. The further pursuit of this knowledge might not only impact on the anti-D debate but also on the experience of childbearing women in general.

CHAPTER NINE

Positive intercessions

As well as discussing the aspects of modern birth felt to cause rhesus isoimmunization, midwives also raised the idea of a number of 'positive intercessions' that may help protect a woman from fetomaternal haemorrhage and the consequences of this. In particular, midwives focused on ways to optimize the health of a woman during pregnancy, with particular reference to naturally strengthening her placenta and immune system. (It should be noted that the word 'positive' is used to denote the addition of these suggestions to the existing body of knowledge in this area rather than being a judgement of the value of such intercessions.)

The term 'intercession' as used by some of those midwives who participated in this study, generally refers to those suggestions that relate to women making positive changes to their diet or lifestyle. It may also involve the use of a naturally occurring substance (such as a herb or essential oil) or another aspect of an alternative therapy (for example yoga, osteopathy or meditation) in order to prevent a problem. An intercession differs from an intervention in several ways; while the former treats a problem, the latter is perceived to be more closely linked to the concept of intercepting and preventing a problem before it requires more aggressive intervention. Further analysis of these differences is shown in Table 9.1. It should be noted that this concept analysis has been derived from the responses of the midwives in this study; it may not be representative of other midwives' understanding.

Table 9.1 Analysis of the differences between intervention and intercession in midwifery

Intervention	Intercession
Usually a medical procedure; sometimes invasive	Not a medical procedure; generally non-invasive
May involve technology and/or pharmaceutical drugs	Doesn't involve technology or drugs; may involve a natural substance, alternative healing modality or lifestyle change
Generally used in order to 'cure' or solve a perceived problem in the body	Works in conjunction with the body to optimize physiological potential
May be used routinely	Always used in relation to the individual woman and her needs
Usually controlled or performed by professionals	Usually controlled by the woman herself
May work against physiology	Works to enhance physiology

It could be argued that, in an historical sense, some intercessions may confer benefit by enabling women to become more aligned with 'nature's original intention'. For example, women deliberately choosing to eat whole or organic foods, or those adopting a vegetarian or vegan diet may be closer to the dietary habits of our ancestors than those women who eat a diet more representative of modern Western lifestyles (Robbins, 1987; Lark, 1999). Often, positive intercessions work towards maximizing the physiological potential of the woman's body and ensuring that medical interventions do not become necessary. Table 9.2 lists the intercessions that midwives felt would help a woman who wanted to avoid the need for anti-D.

Validating midwifery knowledge and evidence

It is interesting to note that the kind of evidence offered in this chapter would, at one time, have been one of the few kinds of evidence available to women or their midwives. Herbal and nutritional lore was passed down many generations of women in general, and

Table 9.2 Positive intercessions that midwives felt might offer protection against isoimmunization

- Optimal nutrition during pregnancy was cited as being of benefit in strengthening the placental bed and reducing the chance of feto-maternal haemorrhage. Midwives felt women should concentrate on eating whole foods, fresh, raw vegetables, pulses and seafood.
- Midwives also suggested that women should avoid substances such as food additives, caffeine and alcohol, which may deplete essential minerals.
- A number of vitamins and minerals are thought to strengthen the placenta; these include magnesium, iodine, vitamin C and bioflavinoids. It was suggested that these could either be incorporated into the diet or taken as a supplement.
- It was suggested that fluoride interferes with the formation of collagen in the placental wall, and that women should avoid drinking fluoridated water and using toothpaste containing this before and during pregnancy.
- Other pollutants such as xenoestrogens were also mentioned as being detrimental to normal physiology and optimal immune status and therefore best avoided by pregnant women.
- Herbs that are thought to offer a protective element by strengthening the uterus and placenta or having a positive effect on the woman's immune system include red raspberry leaf, elderflower and echinacea.
- Garlic was also offered as a preventative treatment, because of its positive effects on the immune system; again, this could be taken as food or supplement.
- A daily dose of activated charcoal, which is known to absorb toxins, was also offered as an aid to the immune system.
- The avoidance of directed pushing during birth was thought to have a positive effect in reducing maternal and fetal stress and the likelihood of transplacental haemorrhage. Similarly, the use of positions that optimize fetal descent and reduce the perceived need for direction was also thought to be beneficial.
- Following on from the idea that immunosuppression was an important feature in preventing isoimmunization was the suggestion that the hormones released while breastfeeding in the early days may also be a protective mechanism against antibody production.
- Several midwives stressed the importance of the emotional and spiritual aspects of birth and the women's psyche. Although no prescriptive preventative or supportive treatment was offered, it was suggested that midwives should explore this area with women before and possibly during birth in order to 'clear' any issues that may arise and could inhibit normal physiology.

midwives in particular, for the benefit of whole communities. Yet today some of this evidence would be considered 'soft', especially in relation to the so-called 'hard' scientific knowledge preferred by the medical model. Why has this experiential and personal knowledge been rejected in favour of impersonal data that may be meaningful in terms of the population, but not of the individual?

If proponents of the medical model were using only those data that were truly scientific and systematically rejecting those practices that could not be proven beneficial or safe, they may then have more of a case for suggesting that this 'softer' data should not be used in practice. However, this is not the case. Many of the practices that are common features of obstetric departments are not based on 'hard' evidence; indeed, in some cases these practices have already been shown to be harmful when used on a routine basis. This situation raises a dilemma, which on one level concerns the need to ensure that we are doing our best to evaluate the knowledge that we might use in relation to birth, such that we are not suggesting anything that we know not to be safe. Yet don't women have the right to all manner of information, even if this is not considered 'hard', if they are facing difficult decisions? Surely women are able to consider their own choices in the light of what is important to them? The important issue must be that women are aware of the sources of such information, and the potential biases of these sources, rather than being given only the information that those who perceive themselves as 'in control' deem fit for consideration.

With this debate in mind, external sources were sought to further validate some of the information given in this chapter. This is not to imply that the data will not stand on their own, but it will confirm that there is evidence within the pseudoscientific framework favoured by the medical model to support several of the suggestions being made. Interestingly, one of the sources later found to mirror some of the information given in this study was a book written by midwife Anne Frey (1997). Frey had already noted some of the same evidence, although the majority of midwives who took part in this study (including myself) had not read her book prior to it. The fact that these two sources of knowledge were derived independently of each other and yet contain broadly similar information may offer some support for the status of such knowledge.

Finally, just as midwives stressed that some of the suggestions here will not be useful to women on a routine or general basis, but rather only when used in relation to the needs of the individual, it should be remembered that this is the very beginning of a debate in this area and many questions remain unanswered. As discussed in previous chapters, the suggestion that certain substances boost the immune system relates to the important philosophical debate concerning the physiological status of this during normal pregnancy. Does the 'modified immune system' need foods that boost its function? How do particular types of herbs and other foods work with the immune system in pregnancy? Are there times when the immune system is better unstimulated? How does stimulation relate to the process of isoimmunization in the presence of a minute transplacental bleed? These and many other questions are still being debated by midwives.

Nutrition

It is no accident that nutrition is the first factor listed here; it was the intercession discussed most often by the midwives in this study. It is also the aspect of holistic health care in general which seems to make the most difference, yet to be the most ignored, by the majority of those who offer care to pregnant and birthing women.

'Optimal nutrition' to these midwives consisted of the following:

- Whole foods, e.g. whole wheat bread and pasta, brown rice
- Organic foods wherever possible
- Plenty of fibre in the diet
- Lots of fresh vegetables, preferably raw
- Pulses, seeds, nuts, beans and legumes as an alternative to meat
- Some midwives suggested seafood in moderate amounts; others felt that a well-planned vegan diet could be adequate.

Foods midwives suggested women should avoid included:

- Red meat
- Dairy products
- Processed or fried food, or that treated with pesticides.

The suggestion that food links closely with health is by no means a new one. Lark (1999) discusses evidence which suggests that whole grains are excellent sources of phytoestrogens, particularly lignans and rutin, which help to strengthen capillaries and tone the uterus.

Seeds and nuts are a source of prostaglandins, another substance related to naturally occurring female hormones, which help to tone the uterus and may be effective in creating optimum uterine tone and a healthy placental bed (Lark, 1999).

Although there are some who believe that a vegan diet is perfectly adequate for women (Robbins, 1987), Odent, 1996 supports the suggestion that sea foods – particularly those found in coastal areas – may be as important as 'land foods' to some pregnant women. Whatever the individual's preference in this area, all sources of evidence suggest that care should be taken to ensure that women are eating the 'right kinds' of fat (e.g. omega fatty acids) to promote healthy uteroplacental blood flow (Odent, 1996).

Some midwives pointed out that increasing foods such as vegetables alone might not be helpful if women eat foods that are not organic. The pesticides and other chemicals that may be present in vegetables may cause harm, or at least negate the benefits of an otherwise healthy diet, and choosing organic produce would seem to be the best way of avoiding these.

The second aspect of nutrition that was mentioned concerned substances that may deplete essential minerals, including food additives, caffeine and alcohol. These are substances that have been understood for some time to be harmful (Robbins, 1987), and they have been termed 'anti-nutrients' by Holford (1997), who notes that good nutrition is a combination of avoiding those substances that are harmful while ensuring adequate amounts of beneficial foods. He suggests that the main categories of anti-nutrient foods are refined foods, chemical additives (such as colourings), pesticides, genetically modified foods, and fried food.

Vitamins and minerals

It is well acknowledged that an adequate supply of vitamins and minerals is important during pregnancy, and a few are highlighted here as being especially beneficial in strengthening the placenta: magnesium, iodine, vitamin C and bioflavinoids. Vitamins and minerals are also suggested to be beneficial – in general and in pregnancy – for other reasons; for example, zinc is suggested to improve the function of the immune system (Herb Research Foundation, 1997). This implies that, while there is good reason to consider the effect of specific vitamins and minerals in relation to the prevention of isoimmunization, it may benefit women to increase the amounts of vitamins and minerals in their diet generally. Further research on specific substances might help to determine whether one or more of these is particularly beneficial for rhesus-negative women.

To date, citrus bioflavinoids are the only substances in this group that have been identified and explored in relation to this area. Even before anti-D was tested, these substances had been shown to strengthen placental attachment and increase the strength of blood vessels (Jacobs, 1956, 1960, 1965). The research also showed that these substances could improve the outcomes of babies born to women who had already become isoimmunized. While this research may have been ignored in favour of the more lucrative drug products being developed in this area, the results remain a starting point for midwives to explore the issues further.

One more recent debate concerning vitamins and minerals regards whether it is better to incorporate these in the diet, or to take a regular supplement in addition to a healthy diet. Again there are proponents of each viewpoint, although the evidence does not seem to be overwhelming either way. While there is certainly something to be said for eating a diet containing as much fresh food as possible, it seems futile not to acknowledge the benefit of supplements for those people who cannot eat the way they might always like to because of their lifestyle or job. The bottom line would seem to be the individual's personal needs and preferences.

Avoiding toxins in the environment

The main toxin that midwives suggested should be avoided by rhesus-negative women is fluoride, perhaps because this is one that is commonly encountered by all women who drink water from the tap, or use toothpaste containing this. While fluoride is accepted as being potentially toxic to all of us (Colquhoun and Mann, 1986; Hirzy, 1999), it is seen as a particular danger to pregnant women because it may interfere with the formation of collagen in the placental wall. The evidence collated by Hirzy (1999) suggests that fluoride has a negative impact on bone formation. While it has proven impossible to find studies that specifically report effects of fluoride on placental formation, women and midwives may feel that there are enough parallels between musculoskeletal and placental formation to warrant further consideration of rhesus-negative women's fluoride intake during pregnancy.

There is also an increasing amount of knowledge concerning pollutants such as xenoestrogens, which are also perceived as being detrimental to normal physiology and optimal immune status. Interestingly, much of this information is circulating on the Internet, which appears to have become a significant source of data regarding alternative lifestyles, and therapeutic and potentially pathogenic substances. Safe and Gaido (1998) define xenoestrogens as chemical contaminants which act in much the same way as oestrogens, yet are harmful rather than therapeutic. They contrast with the more helpful, and naturally occurring phytoestrogens. Xenoestrogens are found in plastics, clingfilm and many other industrially produced compounds.

Herbs

A number of herbs are thought to offer protection to rhesus-negative women in that they either strengthen the uterus and/or placenta, or because they have a positive effect on the immune system. Those cited by the midwives in this study include red raspberry leaf, elderflower and echinacea. While there is evidence to support the use of these herbs in pregnancy, and confirmation that they display the beneficial properties cited in controlled trials, it is important to recognize that herbs are powerful substances that can also have undesirable effects. For this reason, it may be seen as more appropriate for this aspect of the evidence to form the starting point for further research by specialists in the field of herbal medicine.

Another reason for not wishing to pursue this question generally in relation to other evidence is that the midwives did not appear to intend that these herbs were taken as a routine measure, but rather that women should be assessed individually in relation to their potential need for such therapies. In this way, a herbalist/midwife would be able to help the woman determine what was right for her rather than suggesting a universal blend of herbs that would be no more specific to the individual woman's needs than is the average pharmaceutical headache pill.

Garlic

Garlic is also well known as a substance that has positive effects in strengthening the immune system and it was also suggested here as a preventative treatment for rhesus-negative women wishing to reduce the risk of transplacental haemorrhage. Garlic is known to contain a number of minerals, and is particularly high in selenium; a mineral that stimulates the immune system and also bears anti-oxidant properties (Thrash and Thrash, 1981). As with the vitamins and minerals discussed above, garlic can either be included in the diet or taken as a supplement.

Charcoal

Charcoal has been used as a natural remedy throughout recorded history, although its use has decreased since the advent of pharmaceutical drugs (Thrash and Thrash, 1988). This is not because its effectiveness has decreased, but most likely as a result of market forces; charcoal remains cheap to produce and easy to administer, thus there is little money to be made from marketing charcoal products. Because of its massive surface area to volume ratio it can adsorb many times its own weight in toxins or potentially toxic substances, and is the treatment of choice for many practitioners when faced with poisoning or other intestinal disorders (Cooney, 1980).

Because of its potency as a clinical adsorbent, midwives have suggested that charcoal may be a useful substance for rhesus-negative pregnant women to take in order to remove toxins and support the functioning of their immune system. Although some midwives suggested a 'daily dose', there is no optimum amount; yet again, the key is that a woman should look at her personal needs, health, diet and lifestyle, and, in conjunction with her midwife, decide on the amount and frequency which is best for her. Certainly it is widely recognized that moderate amounts of charcoal can 'do no harm' (Thrash and Thrash, 1988) and, in conjunction with good nutrition, this may well be a useful aid to avoiding negative effects of toxins on the immune system during pregnancy.

Avoiding directed pushing

The avoidance of directed pushing during birth was considered by the midwives in this study to have a positive effect in reducing maternal and fetal stress and the likelihood of transplacental haemorrhage. This is a suggestion that has already been discussed. Some of the issues concerning the differences between directed and spontaneous pushing were presented in Chapter 7; currently, it would seem better for women experiencing uncomplicated births to push spontaneously, in order to prevent unnecessary trauma.

In terms of positive intercessions, the midwives had a follow-on suggestion; that the use of positions that optimize fetal descent would be beneficial in reducing the need for pushing generally. This is echoed by Sutton (2000), whose work with midwives and women highlights the differences between a truly physiological second stage and the kind of second stage that women often experience when they choose hospital based or medically managed birth. In physiological second stage, women tend to adopt positions that are upright, forward-leaning and open; this optimizes the position of the baby in relation to the woman's body and may well impact on physiology at this time. Certainly the only advantage in women lying or sitting on beds to give birth is that this affords the person catching the baby a better view of what is happening.

Breastfeeding

Following on from the idea that immunosuppression may be an important feature in preventing isoimmunization was the suggestion that the hormones released while breastfeeding in the early days may also be a protective mechanism against antibody production. A number of questions concerning the existence and nature of immunosuppression in pregnancy were raised in Chapter 7; until we have begun truly to debate the physiological state of the immune system in pregnancy, any discussion of related issues could be somewhat premature.

The fact that the midwives seemed to see the whole of the childbearing year as inter-related and symphonic illustrates their view that all aspects of pregnancy, birth and the postpartum period are interlinked. Within the midwifery model, breastfeeding is seen as a natural, integral and important aspect of the childbearing period; as such, it is not outside the bounds of possibility that breastfeeding is somehow involved in the natural and physiological protective mechanisms which are thought to be available to rhesus-negative women.

Emotional and spiritual health

Finally, several midwives stressed the importance of emotional and spiritual aspects of birth and the women's psyche. Although no prescriptive preventative or supportive treatment was offered, it was suggested that midwives should explore this area with women before and possibly during birth in order to 'clear' any issues that may arise which could inhibit normal physiology or somehow 'block' an aspect of the birth process.

Embracing the innate spirituality of birth is not a new concept; this age-old idea was revisited in modern times by Gaskin (1977), whose data highlighted the advantages of creating an atmosphere where midwives are open to the various spiritual energies of birth and the needs of mother and baby. Eason (1999) documents mothers' experiences of communicating with their unborn children, and highlights evidence that supports the suggestion that women can develop and grow through pregnancy, perhaps by tapping into these intuitive processes. Anecdotally, more midwives are realizing that spirituality is important to women and finding ways of bringing this into their own practice.

Implications for the antenatal anti-D debate

The question of whether fetomaternal haemorrhage is really 'silent' has been raised a number of times already. While the data presented in this chapter do not relate to specific indicators for transplacental haemorrhage, they do beg the question of whether this is preventable, even in a proportion of women, by changes in a woman's diet or lifestyle. This does not simply relate to postnatal transplacental haemorrhage, but may also have implications during the antenatal period, perhaps offering protection against the possibility of antenatal transplacental haemorrhage. These intercessions constitute relatively simple and economical measures that may be found to offer protection without the attendant risks of antenatal anti-D for women who wish to avoid this.

It has already been noted that much of this evidence is new to the area and that, as such, it has not been tested within a quantitative framework. Some of the data contained herein may be a springboard for further research. While this would be the ideal outcome in relation to the standard scientific model of testing such hypotheses, some women and midwives may consider that elements of these data, such as nutritional advice, are 'safe' enough to be incorporated into their routines without further confirmation of efficacy. This is more a reflection of the needs of some women in relation to this intervention than their feelings generally about health research.

Certainly, it is not being suggested that these intercessions form any kind of an 'answer' to the current issue. We are only beginning to debate this complex area, both on philosophical and practical levels. Some of the ideas presented in this chapter may be found to be useful, either generally or to a specific group of women. There may be other as yet unmentioned intercessions that mitigate the changes of isoimmunization; we need to remain open to these possibilities. We also need to consider, on a wider level, what kinds of evidence we can and do use in midwifery practice, and how this evidence can be evaluated and validated in order to help more women and babies.

CHAPTER TEN

Supporting women making decisions

Women should be the focus of care and enabled to make informed choices.

The final theme of the midwifery data concerned midwives' desire and need to support women in making informed choices about their care. The responses that formed this theme covered a variety of issues, which will be outlined before considering the concept of informed choice in this area in more depth.

The pros and cons of anti-D: telling women's stories

As part of the more general theme of 'supporting women's choice', midwives focused on the experiences of women who had received or declined anti-D. The vast majority of midwife participants gave examples of clinical situations they had encountered in this area, and their responses were overwhelmingly grounded in the experiences and needs of the women they worked with. This served both to complement the more philosophical data and to confirm that they were well placed to comment on these issues. Some told the stories of women who, after consideration of the issues, declined anti-D:

> I cared for a Rh-negative primipara who produced a rhesus-positive baby. She managed her own physiological third stage. The lab assays showed no evidence of fetal cells in the maternal circulation 3 hours after birth. {She did not receive anti-D}. I

will hopefully be following this woman through her next pregnancy and will be able to see if any sensitization occurred through routine pregnancy antibody screening.

As well as giving details of women who had declined anti-D, midwives also documented cases where they wondered whether this had caused harm to recipient women:

> I had a client ... who was A negative. When I did her routine {antenatal} lab work, they say she's A positive. Re-did it twice = A+. She had received rhogam with other two pregnancies (different doctors, different cities). After her beautiful home birth with me, she developed toxic shock. Was this a coincidence? Or was the administration of rhogam perhaps partly at fault? I am not sure, even though I understand the mechanism of rhogam.

There is more than one possible explanation for this occurrence; while it may be that this woman had a weak form of the rhesus antigen (Du), which was not found on first testing, it could also be that she suffered augmentation or some other unusual occurrence. It seems less important to establish the exact reason for this than to highlight the situations midwives may face in practice and the real need for them to have an in-depth understanding of the issues in order to be able to talk to women about these.

The following quote may appear to offer information that initially seems quite subjective. However, further discussion with the participant revealed that the woman concerned had taken no other drugs prior to or during her pregnancy and labour:

> One of my relatives received rhogam after the birth of her first baby. Immediately after the injection, she developed a rash over her entire body. This lasted for days, and she couldn't even wear clothes because it hurt/itched so much. She was covered in lotion all the time, but nothing relieved it. She is convinced it was the rhogam, because it was a day after the birth and she had not had any other drugs. I think she was right. It's actually a pretty nasty drug.

Although this research explored midwives' views and information was not solicited from childbearing women, voice must be given to all the women who called, e-mailed or wrote to me during this project. Many of these women had obtained my contact details from

British and American consumer organizations with a health or maternity care focus.

Altogether, 19 women made contact during the initial part of this research. All of them were rhesus negative, and most were concerned with the effects of and necessity for anti-D – often because they had experienced unpleasant side effects from a previous dose. Several told me how their immune systems had been moderately or severely compromised after receiving this product, and some were considering not having any more children because of the 'risk' of needing anti-D again. None of the women who contacted me felt that they had received adequate information from their caregivers – this was often their prime reason for seeking further information – and several stated that they did not even realize that they had a 'choice' in this area until afterwards.

One of the most important questions that midwives must ask is whether or not women are aware that anti-D is a blood product. In my own experience, and that of other midwives approached, most women who are told they might need a blood transfusion (perhaps because their haemoglobin is found to be low postnatally) will question whether this is truly necessary. Even those who do not have a philosophical or spiritual objection to this and who may not have questioned other interventions in their pregnancy and birth are often reluctant to accept a blood transfusion unless this is deemed to be vital. One of the main reasons for this seems to be that women are aware of the potential for virus transmission. I have seen women with symptomatic anaemia who preferred to experience the fatigue this caused rather than receive donated blood, and this experience is not unique.

However, it is a rare woman who questions her need for anti-D in the same way. Why does this discrepancy occur? While it could be argued that this is a reflection of the importance women place on anti-D in protecting their subsequent children, this seems to be a less logical assumption than that women simply do not know that anti-D is a blood product. If they did, probably more would question their need for this in the same way that they do for other blood products. The fact that anti-D is a yellow fluid that comes in a syringe rather than a red fluid in a bag labelled 'blood' should perhaps make us even more aware of the need to discuss this issue with women. The question of whether women's fears in relation to blood (or blood products) are based on sound evidence is less relevant at this time than whether those women are consenting to the administration of a product without prior knowledge of its composition.

In a review of a previous article on this subject, midwife Mary Stewart (1999) wrote:

> I thought back to the times I have talked about anti-D with women and realized that these conversations have not allowed room for real two-way discussion. My input has been along the lines of: 'Well, you are rhesus negative. If you have a rhesus-positive baby, you will need anti-D'. Absolutely no informed choice there, I am ashamed to admit.

I suspect Mary speaks for a number of midwives, and it is not my intention that midwives should feel ashamed; there is no suggestion that midwives fail to inform women out of malice, but perhaps because they are not aware of the issues themselves. Busy midwives may not always have the time to read up on every aspect of the care they offer, and the present culture of maternity care does not make this a priority. Even if midwives do possess the requisite knowledge, constraints in practice often make it difficult for them to spend enough time talking with individual women about their options. It is very difficult in the current climate of sparse resources and midwife shortages to sit with every rhesus-negative woman and explain the risks and benefits, pros and cons of anti-D to her.

Perhaps the most salient issue is that of 'hospital policy'; as long as maternity units have policies (even those couched as guidelines) which midwives are expected to follow, then those midwives who offer the 'whole story' to women run the risk of having those women question their need for anti-D, or even decline its administration. This may then lead to the midwife being questioned, and potentially labelled as a troublemaker:

> I was made to feel so responsible, as if it would've been my fault if the woman had had a problem {after refusing anti-D}. How can we facilitate choice if we don't get the support to do that? Even the women who do want to take responsibility don't seem to be able to get that. Instead, it's the midwife who gets the hassle, while the woman is talked to like a naughty little girl.

This situation may come to parallel that which currently occurs in many units when women decline to have vitamin K administered to their healthy baby. In the case of vitamin K, the choice may be simpler; analysis of the research suggests that this is not necessary for the vast majority of babies, and it is easier to be clear about which babies may benefit from it. Yet it is the policy in a number of units that, when a woman declines vitamin K, her midwife is expected to report or document this. In some units, the refusal of vitamin K will lead to a paediatrician being called to speak to the woman and attempt to talk her out of her choice 'for the sake of the baby'. A number of women are intimidated enough by this practice to change their minds, and subsequently agree to the administration of vitamin K. If women's choices are not respected in relation to vitamin K, how can we believe that they will be in the case of anti-D, which may be deemed equally (or even more) necessary within the medical model?

While the issues are complex and the situation often difficult for midwives, who are at the front line of maternity care, the fact remains that women have a right to make informed choices about their care. Administering a product to women without informing them fully of its composition, potential side effects or other relevant issues is a contravention of professional and ethical codes. At present, there is no legal precedent for a midwife or doctor to be sued as a result of administering such a product without fully informed consent, but this fact should not be seen as protective or reassuring by birth attendants. Legal action could be taken at any time, and anyone who does not enable fully informed choice is potentially at risk of standing trial in a test case.

While defensive and intervention-led practice by health professionals appears to have evolved historically through the fear of being sued for not acting or intervening where a choice existed, the tide now seems to be turning. It is becoming almost as likely that health professionals will be at risk if they do act without fully informing women (and patients) and gaining written consent. How long will it take us to respond to this? Or will we continue to ask women to sign disclaimers only when they decline such interventions, while failing to ensure that women have the most accurate and up-to-date information upon which to base their decisions?

Enabling informed choice

Midwives were very specific about the nature of the information they felt women should be able to expect from their caregiver about anti-D:

> I make sure that women are well informed regarding the impli-cations of their rhesus status related to pregnancy and birth {and} the recognition of the possibility of future sensitization and the potential hazards associated with using human blood products. In other words, the advantages and disadvantages of preventative health care related to the Rh project.

> Women need all of the available evidence provided in a manner which enhances their understanding and retention of such knowledge. Verbal explanations should be given at the level of comprehension necessary. Explanations can be reinforced with printed articles, research abstracts, referrals to other references, depending on the woman's need for knowledge.

Midwives also noted that some women were keener to challenge the *status quo* regarding anti-D than others, regardless of what their usual practice was in trying to enable informed choice in this area:

> ... with people who like to live as close as possible to having 'control' of their lives, I offer them the option, and they often choose to have rhogam, although it costs US$100 (the equiva-lent of £60).

> It depends on her philosophy, her ideas about birth and spiri-tuality. Some women want to talk about it, and have me help decide what it best for them, but others are just like, well do most people have it?

Another midwife agreed that, in her experience, women often fol-lowed the *status quo*, adding the following comment:

> Well 'most people' eat red meat, but that doesn't mean it's good for you!

This highlights an interesting point; what if the woman elects not to choose, but prefers the caregiver or institution to make the decision for her? In many ways, this is what happens now for most women in relation to anti-D. Is this professionally or ethically justifiable? While the ethical debate will no doubt continue, we surely have a professional responsibility to make women aware that there is hardly ever only one viewpoint in midwifery (particularly in the areas where this is practised alongside obstetrics). For the vast majority of women, the philosophy of the caregiver or institution creates the 'norm' and will influence women's decisions. How can we enable more women to become aware of this and to decide what they believe for themselves? Further to this, can we help women to see that the norms they face during childbearing are shaped by the pervasive cultures of technological society, capitalist values and the mass media?

Consistently, the midwives believed women should be informed of the issues and offered whatever information was available, whatever the constraints or barriers to this in practice. Although in theory the medical paradigm seeks informed consent from women before any intervention, in practice the assumption may be made that, by attending for care, the woman is consenting to those interventions that her attendants deem necessary. The difference in the midwifery paradigm was that respondents felt that the choice in this area ought to be explicitly offered to women, along with its pros and cons:

> We don't seem to feel able to tell women this is a choice, to even raise the question of not having anti-D, maybe because we are scared that the potential consequences of a woman declining this choice will be so huge. But it just comes back to the fear stuff – we need to look again at things like who is really taking responsibility here. I think not expecting women to make decisions feeds straight back into the power stuff.

Needing to accept risks

Finally, several midwives discussed the concepts of 'risk' and 'responsibility' as they related to women's birth decisions. The general feeling was that a change in societal attitudes was needed in relation to birth, although most midwives focused on the need to 'work with' individual women. They felt it vital to note, and inform women, that there may never be a total guarantee of protection in relation to isoimmunization:

> I know one woman who had a natural third stage, no intervention. But she still got isoimmunized. This is one in about 25 who declined it. Maybe I'm awful, but I don't think it was a ter-

rible thing, and neither did she. Figured Mother Nature was saying 'enough babies now'.

Women – well, and men – need to accept that there is always an unknown element in birth. Who says, 'nature has the final say'? I can't remember, anyway, that's what I mean, I always say there are no guarantees either way. You might get sick from rhogam, or you might get antibodies without. And the chances of either – well, with physiological birth and a good midwife – are probably pretty small. Much as I would never have rhogam myself, I can see why some women do. But, as I said, I think the most important thing is to look at the way birth is going, I mean in general, and kind of say to women, 'It's your choice, but you do have to think about it and you do have to choose. Take responsibility'. That's the only way we'll get birth back for women.

Enabling informed choice in practice

The remainder of this chapter is devoted to a summary of the information that midwives may want to offer to women and reflection upon how midwives can help women make informed choices in this area. The following points have already been established:

- Around 90 per cent of rhesus-negative women who give birth to a rhesus-positive baby will not need postnatal anti-D. While we can make educated guesses about which women will need anti-D, we have no accurate way of determining this at present.

- Anti-D may cause side effects in some women. As well as those that are generally listed, some evidence emerged in this study to suggest that these may also include immune system compromise. The risk of blood-borne viruses is still under debate. There has been no research into the long-term side effects of anti-D in women, or the long-term effects of antenatal anti-D on women or babies.

- The question of whether or not a woman will want to have anti-D is a complex one, and the key issue may be her personal philosophy.

- Generally, the women for whom this decision will be clear-cut are those who already have strong feelings, either about the normality of the birth process, the product itself, or their desire to have a large family.

- There are no absolutes or guarantees with this decision; a woman who receives anti-D may find that this has not been effective or that she experiences side effects. Equally, a woman who declines anti-D following a physiological pregnancy and birth may find she has developed antibodies.

In terms of women's pregnancy and birth choices, the following has been proposed:

- Women who wish to decline anti-D should carefully consider whether they will consent to medical intervention in their pregnancy and birth (see Chapter 7).

- Women who do undergo interventions during pregnancy and birth, but especially during the third stage of labour, may be more prone to potential isoimmunization. Medical intervention in birth may cause some women's need for anti-D.

- Some midwives believe there are things a woman can choose to do during pregnancy and birth to decrease her likelihood of needing anti-D (see Chapter 9); while these aspects require further research, midwives and women may wish to reflect upon the information given.

There are also points at which the woman can gain clinical information concerning her need for anti-D, if she so chooses:

- Kleihauer testing, while not 100 per cent accurate in ruling out transplacental haemorrhage, may tell a woman if she has experienced this, thus enabling her to decide whether or not to have anti-D. This can be carried out at any time during pregnancy if a bleed is suspected, or in the first few days following the birth.

- There are also a number of clinical signs that midwives may find useful in determining whether or not transplacental haemorrhage has occurred (see Chapters 7 and 8); a few women have been happy to make an 'educated guess' in the light of an inconclusive Kleihauer.

- Where women do not want to receive anti-D, a blood test can be performed later, which will tell them whether they have developed antibodies. This may be helpful for women who do not want anti-D under any circumstances, but who wish to decide upon this evidence whether to become pregnant again. Once antibodies have formed, there is no way these can be removed; pregnancy following antibody formation may require medical intervention.

- There are also tests that will check the woman's partner's blood type; women who know their partner is rhesus negative will not even need to consider antenatal anti-D, or whether they need anti-D if they miscarry. If a woman's partner is rhesus positive, testing can also determine whether he is homozygous or heterozygous rhesus positive. A woman who has a partner who is homozygous rhesus positive will always have rhesus-positive babies; if he is heterozygous rhesus positive there is a 25 per cent chance that each baby will be rhesus negative. It should be noted that these tests may not be routinely available, and that women may need to argue for their right to have them undertaken, or alternatively pay for the tests themselves.

It is almost impossible for any health attendant to offer a woman completely unbiased information on any decision she might need to make. Whatever the issue, we all have our own opinions and experiences, and work within guidelines and resource bases. This cannot help but influence the choices open to women, and the way we frame these for them. We may seek to reassure a woman that she does not really need a screening test which she would have to pay for herself and cannot afford, although she might have a distant family history of a particular problem. We might also find it difficult to be open with women about 'alternative' choices if we are practising in an environment where the philosophy of the system or our colleagues overtly or covertly opposes those choices. It is extremely difficult for anyone to remove all of those influences when framing a decision for a woman.

One of the ways of dealing with this is openly to state our bias and remind women that lots of people have different opinions. When talking to women about vitamin K, for instance, one of the first things I do is to tell them how I personally feel, and so ask them not just to hear my views, but to seek out someone who thinks and feels differently about it. I then go on to explain that there are two ways of looking at the situation, and explain each of the viewpoints involved.

In the case of vitamin K, the viewpoints are clear; the medical model suggests that all babies have low levels of vitamin K and therefore need this to prevent a potentially serious condition. On the other hand, proponents of the midwifery model may feel that babies are born with everything else they need, so why not vitamin K as well?

Research is also suggesting that the latter viewpoint is gaining more support. By outlining and explaining each of these models, and the basic philosophy on which they are based (in whatever terms are most appropriate for the individual woman), it becomes easier for a woman to understand the choice presented and, perhaps more importantly, why she may receive conflicting advice from professionals, friends and the media.

It may be possible to use the same type of presentation with regard to anti-D; the two models present differing perspectives, based on contrasting ethical and philosophical belief systems. We can stress that there are things which are certain (that anti-D is beneficial, that anti-D is not necessary for the majority of women) and things that are uncertain (the risk of side effects, an exact way of working out who will become isoimmunized without anti-D). When we can be honest with women about our own motives, experience and philosophy, then maybe we can offer information which, if not totally unbiased, at least enables the woman to 'see where we are coming from' and place this in relation to her own beliefs and knowledge.

Whatever we say to women individually, it is clear that we also need to work towards systems which are more honest. We need to find ways of opening this dialogue with colleagues who may not trust women's bodies to give birth, and we need somehow to address the misinformation generated by the media and other societal institutions. We also need to ensure that the cultures in which we work are supportive of women making 'alternative' decisions, and not punitive. We must support those midwives who insist on offering information that is not normally shared with women. Perhaps some of the other problems that westernized, medicalized societies face today would be solved if we could only find ways to enable women to reclaim the responsibility for their bodies and decisions.

CHAPTER ELEVEN

Midwifery and medical paradigms

Chapter 5 outlined some of the differences between the midwifery and medical paradigms; the data presented in the preceding chapters serve to illustrate these differences and hopefully also to expand the debate concerning any individual woman's need for anti-D. Chapters 2–4 considered the medical evidence and showed that there remain large gaps in our knowledge in this area and, more importantly, in the information we are able to offer women. It can be seen from Chapters 6–10 that the midwives who participated in the midwifery study offered a vast range of both general and specific knowledge and ideas within the 'midwifery model', many of which are new to the field. Certainly they demonstrate a move away from the traditional 'received view' in the area, offering a range of ideas to explain the issues concerned and with a very definite focus on the practicalities of midwifery practice.

To support the theory that anti-D was not necessary on a routine basis, midwives offered explanations for the occurrence of rhesus isoimmunization, as well as suggestions of positive and intercessionary (as opposed to interventionary) ways in which this could be avoided. Participants also held strong views on the way in which routine medical involvement has altered the conceptualization of birth, and argued that the resulting levels of intervention may have increased the scale of the problem. Midwives also offered evidence that suggests that the medical model approach to this area of childbearing may be limited and inappropriate in terms of the information it offers to women.

It was also suggested that society may need to reconsider the way birth is viewed, and that the attitude which holds that 'medicine has all the answers' might be rejected in favour of a paradigm acknowledging the presence and influence of physiology, nature and spirituality in birth. This would be both more realistic and more in keeping with what is currently known about the process of childbearing through the midwifery model.

A vast amount of 'new' knowledge and a number of areas for further exploration were offered by participants; these included ways of preventing, identifying and conceptualizing the issue of rhesus isoimmunization which are, again, grounded within a midwifery (as opposed to a medical) paradigm. Midwives also offered insight into other aspects of the midwifery model and illustrated the importance of individuality, spirituality and personal philosophy in the experience of childbearing and the decision-making processes this entails.

In summary, the results of the study support the existence of a midwifery paradigm and body of knowledge concerning the need for the administration of postnatal anti-D to rhesus-negative women who have given birth to rhesus-positive babies. This midwifery paradigm is grounded in theory and practice, and relates to many aspects of the decisions that women need to make. It also refers and responds to the medical paradigm that has dominated the field for many years. Further to this, midwives demonstrate the existence and use of knowledge above and beyond that currently offered or acknowledged by the medical model.

Evidence from the midwifery and medical models

Analysis of the evidence from the medical research highlighted that, although this showed anti-D to be an effective intervention, there was no evidence that anti-D was necessary on a routine basis. The studies showed that around 10 per cent of women were, at that time, at risk of isoimmunization without anti-D. It is only within the medical paradigm that anti-D is seen as being necessary as a preventative measure for all rhesus-negative women who have given birth to a rhesus-positive baby. The midwives in this study viewed this as an intervention that should be offered to appropriate women, but added that these women should realize that they had a range of choices in this area.

The fact that anti-D offers protection to future babies against rhesus disease may well be seen within the medical model as a justifiable reason to administer this to all women who are perceived to be at risk. However, it can be seen that there are a number of women who do not feel this to be at all justifiable; having weighed up the risks and benefits in relation to their personal philosophy and feelings about birth, they choose not to receive anti-D for whatever reason. These are not only the white, well-educated and middle class women who fit the stereotypical model held by some birth attendants, but women from all walks of life. It is just not possible (and certainly not ethical) to offer information only to those women whom an attendant perceives might want it, while assuming that the rest will be happy to have anti-D regardless. The issue is so grounded in personal philosophy that there is no way we can judge from appearances what any woman's choice in this area might be; the only option is to discuss the issue with women and ask for their preference.

Surely then, we can't continue to turn up at a woman's bedside and offer her a 'little injection to protect her babies' without informing her that we can't tell her for sure that the blood product we are about to offer her is truly safe and without potential side effects? Doesn't she deserve to know that only 10 per cent of women who experience a medically managed birth actually need anti-D, and that, although the evidence is sparse compared to that available for some other interventions, we may now have some insight into which women are more or less likely to need anti-D?

The information presented by the midwives is even more pertinent in relation to the debate regarding antenatal anti-D. It has already been established that, before instigating policies that propose the routine administration of this in the antenatal period, we should further determine the effectiveness of postnatal administration and consider other issues that might be skewing the data. The evidence offered by the midwives, which suggests that more medical interventions than first thought may cause fetomaternal haemorrhage, may be relevant to determining why some women are becoming isoimmunized during this time. Again, is there evidence to suggest that a so-called silent fetomaternal haemorrhage may not be so silent after all? Furthermore, we have a starting point for discussion of those intercessions that may provide protection to women. In the absence of a natural alternative to anti-D at the present time, some of these may be found to be useful to women who would not want to put their unborn baby's health at risk.

In terms of enabling choice, it is clear that a fair proportion of women are not being given the information that would enable them to make an informed decision. At the very least, women should be told that anti-D is a blood product, and that the long-term side effects of this have not been researched. They need information concerning the known side effects, although we must also confess that we don't know how often these occur. They certainly need to know that no research has been carried out into the long-term effects of antenatal anti-D on their unborn baby if they are being offered this product in pregnancy. The bottom line is that we need to make it explicit to women that they have a choice to make in this area, and to be able to offer them the evidence we do have.

Comparing the paradigms

It can be seen that, where proponents of the midwifery model view the process of birth as a natural event which takes on a social and spiritual meaning above the physical, issues surrounding isoimmunization are viewed in a different light from that given by the medical model. Medicalization has caused the issue of rhesus grouping in childbirth to be labelled with a notion of pathology, where midwives see the issue as based in physiology and the decision-making process grounded in a woman's spirituality. The more traditional evidence in this area reflects the continued application of Cartesian dualist theory to the birth process (Ginesi, 1998), which suggests that it is possible to consider issues relating to the physical body without considering the emotions, psychology, spirituality or social situation of the person. Yet the midwifery evidence rejects the idea of separation of the different aspects of birth in favour of a more holistic approach to knowledge as well as to women themselves.

As it is now fairly well understood that this dualist model and a total focus on the physical bears little relation to the dynamic and holistic nature of birth, the evidence gained from this study suggests that the medical research upon which policies concerning anti-D administration are based offers only a small part of the evidence regarding this area. The notion of rhesus incompatibility as a pathological (or even potentially pathological) scenario may be outdated in its usefulness to women.

The midwives in this study also suggested that medical model attitudes and intervention in this area may have exacerbated the issue. The original clinical trial data, collected from a population of women who experienced childbirth within the medical model, may not be accurate in determining the level of rhesus isoimmunization in physiological birth. Anecdotal evidence from midwives who were practising at the time the trials were undertaken supports the fact that managed third stage, episiotomy and other interventions were common, which may have biased the original research.

The question of iatrogenesis may throw a different light on our perceptions of anti-D. If medical intervention could have added to the rate of isoimmunization in the first place, then the addition of anti-D to the range of interventions available in medical birth does not appear as heroic and portentous as advocates suggest. Rather, it could be viewed as a reactionary measure that was needed to counteract other problems that the medicalization of birth caused.

Davis-Floyd (1992) refers to this as the one–two punch; where technology developed to solve one problem leads to the need for further technology to solve problems caused by the first technology. The result of this may be that the pathological conceptualization of birth which this creates or supports was inaccurate in the first place, a theory supported by others researching in this field (Davis-Floyd and St John, 1998).

Some of the midwives in the study took this a step further, suggesting that it was not just the medicalization of birth which may have caused this problem, but that the increasing reliance of technology in society may also have played a part. Examples given included the process of fluoridation of water supplies, which may have led to women having less healthy placental beds, and the effects of environmental pollutants and waste on the immune systems and hormonal balances of otherwise healthy women. Clearly, this issue may be about more than the use of technology in birth; it may be linked to the effects on society and individuals of the use of technology in general.

An overwhelming feeling identified among many of the midwives involved in this research was that we – as in Western society – have been socialized to a point where we have 'lost faith' in the process of birth, instead feeling we need to rely on medical intervention and technology to support and enhance a process which is inherently natural and, in the words of one participant, 'virtually infallible'. That midwives see this issue as linked with the theory of rhesus isoimmunization and the various conceptualizations of this was explicit within the data collected. What needs to be done to address this may be a more difficult question.

What next?

The lack of sound information for women needing to make this difficult decision would suggest that further research and analysis on the subject of anti-D is not only warranted but imperative. A further consensus conference might be a starting point, although it is suggested that this should include not only the experts within the medical community, but also an equal proportion of childbearing women, midwives, and representatives from lay and midwifery organizations such as the Association for Improvements in Maternity Services and the Association of Radical Midwives.

It is not helpful to suggest that further research should be carried out without being explicit about the kinds of research that might be undertaken. When originally embarking upon this research, it was my belief that one of the ways forward in research terms might involve working with a population of women who did not yet have access to anti-D. This would essentially have entailed replicating some parts of the original trials, and would have brought up a number of ethical issues and aspects that might not be fair to the women in the study. However, the data discussed in the midwifery study have raised a number of further research questions that could be carried out more simply and locally. These are outlined below, together with a short discussion as to how research into each might be carried out, with the aim of bringing together evidence from all sources to continue to inform the debate.

What is the rate of transplacental haemorrhage in physiological birth?

This research may not need to be confined to rhesus-negative women. If the laboratory test used to determine whether transplacental haemorrhage had occurred was one of those that picked up the presence of fetal haemoglobin rather than any aspect of the rhesus factor, then rhesus-positive women could be included as well. This would greatly increase the number of women who could participate. Testing blood for transplacental haemorrhage would be carried out before any postnatal anti-D was administered (although it would be inappropriate to include in this study rhesus-negative women who had chosen to receive antenatal anti-D), and so a woman's choice in this area would not affect results. This would also ensure that the study would not prevent women who wanted to receive postnatal anti-D from doing so.

This study could either be carried out solely on women experiencing physiological birth or it could include women who had experienced medical intervention in order to compare the data. However, if the latter was the case, it may be difficult to process the data unless a large number of women were involved because of the number of interventions used and the problem of confounding variables. Because so many interventions may potentially cause fetomaternal transfusion, and because it is rare that a woman experiences only one of these interventions, it may be difficult to separate out the data. It should also be noted that, in such a study, women considered to have experienced 'physiological birth' should have experienced truly physiological birth. Including women in the study whose labours or births had been managed in any way may bias the data and lead to less than accurate results. This almost certainly requires the collaboration of holistic midwives with those who would co-ordinate such a study.

What is the effect of obstetric interventions in pregnancy and labour on the occurrence of transplacental haemorrhage? Do interventions in pregnancy lead to 'silent' fetomaternal transfusion?

Admittedly, there has been some work into this area already; this research has confirmed – among other things – that external cephalic version (Vos, 1967; Stine et al., 1985), Caesarean section (du Bois et al., 1991) and amniocentesis (Blajchman et al., 1974; Lachman et al., 1977) may all increase the likelihood of a woman experiencing transplacental haemorrhage. Further research could be carried out on the other interventions which midwives have suggested could lead to this, whether in the antenatal period or following medically managed labour and birth. Potential problems exist in that women rarely experience only one intervention, and few women currently decline interventions such as ultrasound scans, despite concerns about their safety. Yet this is not an impossible task, and it is precisely this kind of study for which the scientific process used by the medical model is useful. It is also possible that data could be extrapolated from other research into the appropriate interventions and used to inform such a study.

What percentage of women who decline anti-D following physiological birth go on to develop antibodies?

On the basis that there are women who are declining anti-D, inviting these women to participate in a study which looked at the 'true' risk of isoimmunization following physiological birth might help generate this crucial data which would help other women to make their own decisions. From experience, a fair proportion of women who decline anti-D (excepting those who do not plan or are unable to have more children) will have a blood test several months after a birth to determine whether antibodies have formed. It would be a relatively simple matter to collate the results of these blood tests with the data on women's birth experience.

It is acknowledged that, in order to recruit enough women to make the data meaningful, the study would not be geographically based, but might be co-ordinated by one or more researchers to include women from different areas, and even countries. In order to prevent problems of bias, women would need to be recruited during pregnancy and then included or not depending on whether they actually experienced physiological birth and their decision regarding anti-D. The data collection process would need to be designed to include details of the woman's lifestyle, nutritional status and any other aspects of her habits that might be considered as positive intercessions; this might then allow consideration of whether these made a difference.

Do midwifery intercessions (such as nutritional and lifestyle advice) help prevent transplacental haemorrhage/isoimmunization?

While it may not be appropriate at this stage to conduct a study that looked at positive intercessions in preventing transplacental haemorrhage or rhesus isoimmunization, there is great scope for debate in this area. Many questions remain unanswered – even undiscussed by more than small groups of midwives – and this is a relatively new area that may have potential. The questions raised at the end of

Chapter 9 might form the basis for discussion and reflection by midwives, with a view to clarifying the issues for future study. Such study would need to be creatively designed, as the randomized controlled trial approach that generally tests the value of an intervention would clearly not be useful where midwives are suggesting that intercessions need to be specifically chosen to meet the needs of the individual woman.

How do childbearing women feel about the issue of anti-D? What information do women need in order to help them make this decision?

These questions are among the most important, yet are in many ways the most obvious and the easiest to ask. Some excellent feminist research has been carried out in similar areas, and this would seem to be an appropriate approach for an issue that is predominantly of concern to women. I am well aware that, although a lot of women were approached regarding this issue, some of their concerns may have been missed, or other women may feel differently. The research conducted was based firmly within midwifery practice, not women's experience, and a study that looked into this would be extremely useful in conjunction with the midwifery evidence. It is only fair that data from both women and midwives should inform future work in this area.

Can epidemiological data be found to explore the question of environmental effects on rhesus sensitization?

The suggestion that environmental pollution and aspects of modern-day living such as fluoridated water may affect a woman's chance of isoimmunization is relatively new and therefore may be a topic which warrants further analysis with epidemiological and other relevant data. While it would not necessarily be useful to embark on primary research in this area until more is known or surmised about the issues, and perhaps the potential sources of harmful pollution, it would seem foolhardy to ignore this aspect of the data, which echoes that found by other health researchers (Robbins, 1987, 1996; Shelton, 1995). Further collation of data regarding which pollutants may pose a risk to the integrity of the placenta and the immune system would certainly offer more information to women wishing to avoid anti-D. This may also be relevant for other women, such as those who experience problems in pregnancy relating to health of their placenta.

Are there any alternatives to anti-D?

One of the questions uppermost in my mind when this study began was that of whether there was a natural alternative to anti-D, in the same way that there are natural alternatives to many pharmaceutical products, and even homeopathic preparations which are an alternative to immunization. Although the midwifery data revealed the concept of positive intercessions, which could be seen as an alternative in some respects, no alternative product that would reverse the effects of transplacental haemorrhage came to light.

This question is another that begs further philosophical discussion. Nature may well provide substances that restore health and balance in human and animal bodies, yet if isoimmunization is not a feature of physiological birth, then nature may not hold an 'answer'. As with the concept of positive intercessions, the assumptions upon which this question is based need to be unpacked in order to determine whether an answer may be found within the midwifery model or whether the question is rooted in the philosophy of the medical approach. Until that question is debated, it cannot be ruled out that there may be a natural plant or other non-human substance that would act in the same way as anti-D but perhaps be more palatable to those woman who choose not to receive blood products or those containing human immunoglobulin. It would be useful to have more time with the therapists with whom I talked during my research; several of them, although very interested in the issues, had not previously been approached with this question, and needed to do further reading and research of their own in order to formulate an answer. It is hoped that this presentation of the midwifery evidence might trigger discussion of this possibility among those who are experts in health philosophy and alternative therapies.

Funding future research

The issue of research funding is always a difficult one. It is tempting to invite any of the pharmaceutical companies that produce anti-D to offer funding for such research. They are certainly the potential source best placed to offer the amounts required for such work. Yet while it seems only fair that these companies should plough some of their profits back into research that will enable women to base their choices on accurate information, it is the very fact that much of the existing research was funded by these bodies that calls into question its potential validity. Perhaps one answer would be to invite anonymous donations of funds into a trust for further research into anti-D; it would be interesting to see whether such an altruistic and noble opportunity were taken up!

Combining forms of evidence

Ultimately, there are no 'rights and wrongs' regarding philosophical viewpoints, research methodologies and forms of evidence; all have their place in adding to the information women need. All research is flawed in that none can be completely value free, and the fact that analysis may highlight potential biases within the philosophical framework of a research study does not mean that the findings of that study cannot add to our knowledge base. It is simply a case of needing to put research into its philosophical context and exploring all of the evidence and philosophical viewpoints within any given area.

In terms of anti-D, there is certainly a need for further work outside of the medical paradigm that has dominated this field (among many others) for so long. Yet we also need to consider how best to amalgamate the evidence from the medical and midwifery paradigms, together with information from women and any other appropriate sources, into a more useful framework for informing women's decisions and midwifery practice.

CHAPTER TWELVE

Moving midwifery knowledge forward

While the previous chapter considered the differences between the medical and midwifery paradigms and the potential for further research into anti-D, there are yet further issues relating to this and other areas which mainly concern midwives and midwifery evidence. It is these issues that will be considered in this chapter.

Midwifery knowledge

The nature of midwifery knowledge has changed dramatically over history, and it is only within the last few years that midwifery has been influenced by the pseudoscientific knowledge offered by the medical model. Whatever one thinks about the value of scientific and non-scientific forms of evidence, there is no getting away from the fact that, traditionally, midwifery has been more about women's knowledge than men's. It should also be remembered that all knowledge is culturally based and determined. The twenty-first century western world may place a high value on the kind of knowledge that comes from the randomized controlled trial, yet midwives in other cultures and times would not see that this had any relevance to the experience of the women they are with during their births.

In some areas, the art of midwifery has become dominated by medical attitudes, beliefs and knowledge. Yet the voices of the women in this study are clearly holding on to all of the kinds of thought and knowledge they see as valid, despite the fact that many of these may be at odds with the scientifically orientated world in which they live and work. Will we manage to retain this kind of knowledge in mainstream midwifery practice, or will the midwives who have the ability to think, analyse and generate knowledge in this way become increasingly marginalized? An understanding of the development of knowledge and evidence that informs midwifery must surely be pivotal to improving practice and the experience of women.

Women as populations

Analysis of the medical research carried out into anti-D highlights one issue which has influenced the experience of women in this area over the last 30 years. When it was discovered that anti-D was useful for around 10 per cent of women who experienced medically managed birth, the decision was made to administer this to all women. No-one appeared to contemplate the idea that researchers should attempt to determine whether it was possible to tell which women were in the 10 per cent who needed anti-D and which in the 90 per cent who didn't. The professional literature does not even record a debate on this matter.

This issue was also raised by Michel Odent (1999), an obstetrician who is also an expert in birth physiology:

> Try explaining to an intelligent outsider that, for about 30 years, millions of RhD negative women have been routinely injected with an anti-D immunoglobulin when they gave birth or when they had a miscarriage. Explain also that in fact such an injection was not useful for 90% of these women. The intelligent outsider will probably ask what research has been done to determine the 10% who really need anti-D. There is a fundamental incompatibility ... between the art of midwifery and strict protocols which include the word routine. The practice of authentic midwifery presumes that every mother and every baby is a particular case.

How then can we reconcile the practice of individualized 'authentic midwifery' with the use of scientific data which are perceived to be of the most value when gathered from large, homogenous populations?

The problem with routines

Increasingly, midwives and other researchers are carrying out studies that show routine medical intervention in birth not to be a panacea at all, but paradoxical in the context of the physiology of women's bodies. Indeed, it now seems obvious – and well proven – that inappropriate medical intervention in birth is causing far more problems than it is preventing. Has the 'need' for routine anti-D been caused by medical intervention? It is true that rhesus isoimmunization was an issue before the advent of anti-D, but to what degree did the medicalization of birth increase this problem during those decades which spawned so much research into the area? If birth had not become a matter for medical intervention, would rhesus disease have remained an occasional problem, with research focusing on the need to determine which women needed an intervention such as anti-D?

This is not the only example of an intervention that may be iatrogenic; there are many other examples of this within current maternity care. The example of vitamin K is similar in that the need for this has been increased by medical intervention. Generally, the babies who may need vitamin K are those who have traumatic instrumental and operative births, not those who are born physiologically. It is well understood that interventions in labour, such as induction, electronic fetal monitoring, intravenous oxytocin and directed pushing, lead to a 'cascade of intervention' which can result in Caesarean section or instrumental delivery (Kitzinger, 1988; Jowitt, 1993). Studies of women who experience physiological birth, often at home, show that the natural occurrence of real problems in birth is far less than the occurrence of problems following medical intervention, while physiological birth at home is just as safe, and safer in some respects, than medically managed birth in hospitals.

Again, the key seems to be that we need to focus on the individual. There is no answer to the question of whether women 'should' or 'should not' have anti-D. The main reason for this is that the only way this decision should be made is on an individual basis – and the only person who can make that decision is the woman herself.

Exploring and validating midwifery knowledge

One of the major features of the medical model is that it is intrinsically associated with the scientific model of experimentation and investigation (Davis-Floyd, 1992). This model has become the 'gold standard' as far as evidence-based medicine is concerned (Walshe, 1995), and is considered to constitute the authoritative knowledge within our society (Davis-Floyd and St John, 1998). Yet there is movement in the field of evidence-informed midwifery towards the use of evidence other than that generated through the scientific processes.

Midwives use a number of forms of evidence in their work with women, including reflection upon experience, physiology, intuition and common-sense reasoning. These age-old forms of evidence are becoming increasingly accepted as relevant to modern-day mid-wifery (Page, 1997; Edmunds, 1998; Wickham, 1999d). Are the alternative (to quantitative research) types of knowledge that holis-tic midwives use the stepping stones between the data from scientific studies of large populations and the individual women who have to make choices for themselves and their babies?

However, the problem remains that we are only just beginning the debate concerning the measurement and validation of these forms of evidence. While it is important to acknowledge the use of experience and observation in midwifery practice, and the value of the know-ledge we can gain from this, it is equally important to ensure that we are eradicating the trend where attendants are practising in a particular way because of habit or tradition.

Perhaps we need to amalgamate all the different forms of evidence on any given topic, in order to gain a broader picture of knowledge on an issue or aspect of care. This would enable us to ensure that we are utilizing all of the available knowledge in an area, while being able to compare knowledge from different sources. Yet at present there is no generally accepted standard other than the scien-tific model by which to measure or validate the forms of evidence that fall outside the realm and philosophy of this model. This must surely be one of the most pressing needs for midwives to address.

It may be important that we attempt to expand the categories of knowledge open to us, rather than to reduce these by rejecting those forms that do not fit our own philosophy; women have a right to decide which they value for themselves. There remain some ques-tions that we look to the scientific community to answer, which may provide further useful information for women and midwives. Even now, the exact mechanism by which anti-D offers protection against isoimmunization is still not known (Hoffbrand et al., 1999), although several theories have been offered. If we could detail this process and analyse it within the framework of our existing knowledge, we may be even further along the route of discovering which women may be more prone to isoimmunization, or whether there may be a natural alternative to anti-D. Thus, while it is important to consider ways of generating knowledge other than the scientific process, we should also be careful not to 'throw out the baby with the bath water' when it comes to redefining the nature and expanding the role of 'evidence' in midwifery practice.

We also need to think laterally in order to ask the right questions. As discussed in Chapter 11, some of the most stimulating questions in this area remain unexplored. Michel Odent (personal correspondence, March 2000) suggests that we need to explore what the evolutionary advantage of rhesus negativity might be. In the haste to label rhesus negativity with notions of pathology, we have forgotten to ask the simple questions. Along similar lines, Jowitt (1993) raised the question of whether rhesus negativity offered a physiological advantage, in the same way that people with sickle cell anaemia are protected from malaria. Many equally interesting questions remain in this area, some of which have been generated from the data gathered in this study.

The fact that the midwifery study in this area generated such a large and varied amount of data – much of which provided 'new' knowledge – would seem to support the proposition that similar studies might be carried out in other areas as part of a wider exploration of midwifery knowledge. The data collected were rich, explicitly related to midwifery practice, and of a depth rarely found in textbooks or quantitative research articles. Midwives clearly possess and use knowledge from and within another paradigm that I would suggest is far broader than that of the medical model.

This is not an isolated example; there are a number of other sources of this kind of knowledge. A number of midwifery journals continue to publish more traditional forms of midwifery knowledge, such as birth stories, discussion of practice, sharing of alternative remedies, philosophical and reflective articles, and more creative, artistic forms of knowledge. Another key source of this kind of midwifery knowledge can be found on the Internet, a tool which midwives practising in different areas – and sometimes in isolation – have harnessed as a way of discussing practice, problems and solutions with each other. Several web sites have been created to store some of these discussions (see Huntley, 1999), and they hold rich data for those interested in exploring evidence other than that generated through quantitative research.

Midwifery knowledge is currently a neglected area that has been overshadowed in recent times by the focus on obstetric and medical knowledge, although there is clearly massive potential to develop the area further. There is such a vast range of knowledge that falls outside the remit of scientific study that to continue to ignore this would be detrimental to all of us. The implication of not continuing to gather this kind of data may be that we will compound the situation we currently find ourselves in, where this midwifery knowledge may be lost in the face of the pervasive medical paradigm. We need to propose and develop systems and networks to explore this knowledge, along with tools for considering its validation and application in practice. There is clearly room for midwives to explore means of generating knowledge other than through scientific research, and this must be considered a priority for midwives.

Implications for midwifery practice, education and research

The results of this study generate a great deal of new knowledge for consideration and reflection by midwives. Currently, the information that is generally offered to women in this area is limited to that offered by and through the medical model, and the implication of this is that women may not be receiving enough information upon which they can base a truly informed choice. However, this is only the groundwork for such reflection; midwives need to continue to debate these issues and to explore other knowledge within the midwifery paradigm that might help women who face such decisions.

There are many different starting points for women, and this needs to be taken into account when considering the value of different aspects of knowledge on the subject. Some women will want anti-D regardless of any potential risks; they still need to be informed of these in order that they are giving informed consent for its administration. Other women will wish to avoid anti-D, and may want to know how to maximize their chances of avoiding isoimmunization; these women will need information that will enable them to make the choices which are right for them. The majority of women may well fall between these extremes, and it is these women who may find the decision the most difficult. Yet it is these very women for whom the medical profession has been making decisions for the last 30 years. No doubt some midwives will find they need more information themselves in order to help these women; the fact that this is a challenge should not detract from the fact that it should become a priority for those midwives and other attendants who work with rhesus-negative women.

Midwives might also consider the nature of the information and evidence upon which they rely in practice, and reflect upon the current attitude of unquestioned acceptance of the dominance of the scientific and medical models. This study evidences – again – that not only are these models simply one part of the myriad evidence relating to and informing birth decisions, but that they are by no means infallible and without consequences for women and babies. There is overwhelming evidence to support the proposal that all midwives should be exploring other forms of knowledge, and I would suggest that such discourse is well overdue.

One of the features of this study is that the majority of the midwives who participated are based largely in practice; although some are involved in midwifery education to a small degree, this is not the focus of their work. The implication of this is that practising midwives do hold an immense amount of knowledge that is relevant to others, and that research and academia are not the only ways of generating such thought and knowledge. This must be recognized by those who manage midwives, who often fail to provide time for the pursuit of reflective discussion and dialogue.

It is also apparent that, as a society, we actually know very little about the physiology of birth, not least because this has been ignored or usurped in some cases by medicalization of the birth process (Ginesi, 1988). In general, we have probably lost more knowledge about the physiology of birth than we currently hold, and perhaps now is the time to acknowledge this relative lack of knowledge and consider the need to focus on this area in order to improve the outcomes and the experiences of birth for women and babies.

There is something of a paradox involved in presenting research that suggests research should not be the only form of valid enquiry and knowledge generation used to inform midwifery. This debate also requires urgent attention by midwives, particularly those involved in education, academia and research. While this is not to reject the value of the scientific and medical models in their place, we need to be very clear about the nature of their 'place' within the wider framework of evidence that informs midwifery. Concurrently, we need to develop tools to analyse and evaluate other forms of knowledge. As above, it is clearly unacceptable within current standards of care to base practice on knowledge that may be inaccurate or grounded only in tradition or habit. Yet at the same time there is a need to seek and embrace new knowledge that does not fit into current paradigms, and to formulate tools for the evaluation of this knowledge as it relates to midwifery practice.

I would suggest that this debate needs to occur on socio-political as well as personal and practice levels; the overarching dominance of the medical model in birth and midwifery has built up over time, but is now more widely recognized as inaccurate and potentially harmful to women and babies. Yet western society remains captivated by the values of the medical and scientific models, and it is only the occasional woman who feels brave or angry enough to challenge the system. Women need to be offered the evidence from the midwifery paradigm, in order that this can inform their choices. Perhaps the biggest dichotomy here is that many midwives are unwilling to push their views and knowledge about the superiority of physiological (as opposed to medical) birth for fear of biasing women's choices. But women's choices are continually biased by the all-pervasive medical model, which has no doubts of its superiority, even in the light of overwhelming evidence that would dispute this.

The need for the anti-D debate to continue amongst midwives cannot be overemphasized – these data should only be considered a starting point, although it is hoped that they may be useful in highlighting the different paradigms for women and their midwives. As far as the wider debate concerning midwifery knowledge is concerned, we should consider the work of groups of women such as Belenkey et al. (1997), who challenged the value of the seminal – and male – work in their area in relation to women's experiences. This particular group of women talked to women about the ways they learned, and highlighted that 'women's ways of knowing' differed from men's. Not only do their methods illustrate the one woman-centred direction that other researchers could take; their results also offer insight into the ways in which women combine the more rational and scientific forms of knowledge with intuitive and subjective wisdom in order to understand the world around them. Again, the conclusion seems to be that we need inclusive, rather than exclusive, models of midwifery knowledge and evidence.

A final reflection

During this study, I was constantly awed by the level of knowledge and experience that the midwives in this study possessed, but perhaps even more awed by their ability to process their knowledge and experience within the philosophical and reflective frameworks which they had developed.

Davis-Floyd and St John (1998) describe four increasingly open stages of cognitive processing, where 'stage-four thinkers' have the most neural links in their brain and are able to process diverse and new information and link this within the pathways of knowledge they already hold. This might be considered the epitome of an 'open mind'. They see traditional medical systems of knowledge as generally more 'closed', and I would suggest that the nature of the thinking demonstrated by the midwives in this study epitomizes the more open thinking needed to process the many questions with which reflective questioning always leaves us. Perhaps only this type of approach and perspective allows consideration of the 'other side of the story', in contrast to the passive acceptance which has characterized the practice of those midwives and others who have subscribed to medical theories in this area without question.

I am left with the conclusion that the decision regarding anti-D is by no means an easy one for women to make. Indeed, it has become even more complex than before, while at the same time becoming simpler when approached from a personal philosophical perspective. At the onset of this study, I wondered if anti-D was the exception to the general rule that no intervention was necessary on a routine basis in birth. However, this research has showed that anti-D is not an exception to this rule at all, and the midwives have helped demonstrate that there could be no exception to this rule within a midwifery paradigm which sees birth as a natural and spiritual process. There can and should be nothing routine about a rite of passage that is respected as such.

Glossary

ABO incompatibility Describes the situation where a woman is blood type O, while her baby has blood type A, B or AB. Generally, the anti-A or anti-B substances contained in the type O mother's blood may cross the placenta and break down some of the baby's red blood cells, causing jaundice within the first 24 hours. While this is normally not a pathological occurrence, the existence of ABO incompatibility between mother and baby may be relevant in relation to women's need for anti-D.

Anaphylaxis A severe condition of sudden onset which usually follows ingestion of a substance to which the person is severely allergic. This can also occur as a result of receiving a blood product; in this case the person reacts to a component in the blood. The victim's throat can constrict, thereby inhibiting breathing, and the condition requires immediate emergency treatment. Also known as anaphylactic shock.

Antenatal Pertaining to pregnancy. The antenatal period spans the time from when a woman becomes pregnant until she goes into labour.

Anti-D Describes an antibody which may be produced in the blood of a rhesus-negative person who has come into contact with the rhesus 'D' antigen. The antibody would then fight off any further 'D' antigen it encountered in the future. This term also refers to a manufactured product which is administered to prevent the body forming antibodies to the rhesus antigen, where there is concern that this antigen has entered the body.

Antibody	A substance that forms in the body in response to the introduction to an antigen or toxin which enables the body to build immunity to that antigen or toxin in the future.
Antigen	Any substance that enters the body and triggers a reaction which stimulates the immune system to produce antibodies that would protect against the entry of the same antigen in the future.
Controlled cord traction (CCT)	An intervention used to deliver the placenta in a managed (medical) third stage. Once an oxytocic drug has been given to make the uterus contract, the attendant pulls on the placenta to remove this from the uterus. It is suggested that this may lead to an increased chance of feto-maternal haemorrhage as, along with the use of oxytocic drugs, it disrupts the normal physiology of the third stage of labour.
Coombs test	A test which detects antibodies in the blood. A Coombs test may be direct, where it detects antibodies in the baby's blood (as taken from the umbilical cord), or indirect, where the test is carried out on the woman's blood.
Curettage	An operative procedure where a surgeon scrapes the lining of the uterus to remove tissue.
Doula	A woman who is trained and/or experienced in supporting other women during labour or around the time of birth.
Endogenous	The form of a chemical substance which is produced in the body; endogenous oxytocin describes oxytocin which is produced physiologically by the woman's body (cf. exogenous).
Episiotomy	A cut made into the perineal skin between the vagina and the anus just before the birth of a baby.

Exogenous	The form of a chemical substance which is synthetic and introduced into the body; exogenous oxytocin, although similar to that produced by the woman's body, is a synthetic form of the chemical introduced by injection or intravenous drip.
External cephalic version (ECV)	A procedure where an attendant attempts to turn a breech baby so that the head (rather than the bottom) engages in the mother's pelvis. Where this is performed under medical supervision, the procedure involves the attendant placing her hands on the woman's abdomen and manipulating the baby from the outside. This is often performed in conjunction with ultrasound. It should be noted that some holistic midwives have developed a form of ECV which is potentially less invasive.
Extrapolate	To use information or facts known about one area in order to make suggestions relating to another area.
Fetomaternal transfusion	Describes the passage of fetal blood into the maternal circulation at the site of the placenta. This term is used interchangeably with 'transplacental haemorrhage'.
Gamma globulin	The proteins in blood plasma which contain antibodies or immunoglobulins, and may give the recipient passive immunity against disease.
Gene	One unit of the factors that may be passed on from parent to child during the process of reproduction. Genes are located on chromosomes, and each may be dominant or recessive. The genes from the parents will combine, and half of the original genes from each parent will be passed on to each child.
Grounded theory	A qualitative research philosophy and method which uses data collected from people in the 'real world' to build a

	theory or set of ideas around the topic under study.
Haematologist	An expert in the nature, physiology and diseases of blood. A haematologist may be a scientist or a physician.
Haemolytic disease of the newborn	See Rhesus haemolytic disease of the newborn.
Heterozygous	Describes a person who carries two different genes rather than two which are the same. Some rhesus-positive people will carry one gene that is rhesus positive and one that is rhesus negative. Because the gene for being rhesus positive is dominant, people who are heterozygous rhesus positive will always be rhesus positive themselves, but they may pass the rhesus negative gene on to their children.
Homozygous	Describes a person who has a pair of genes which are the same. Rhesus-negative people are always homozygous rhesus negative, because if one of their genes was rhesus positive this would dominate the rhesus-negative gene and they would be rhesus positive instead. A person who is homozygous rhesus positive will always pass a rhesus-positive gene to their children and they will all therefore be rhesus positive.
Iatrogenic	A disease, problem or condition caused by medical, surgical or pharmaceutical intervention.
Immunity	The resistance built up or held by the body to certain specific diseases, tissues, toxic or non-toxic substances or antigens. There are several different kinds of immunity; acquired immunity is produced specifically in response to an antigen, such as the rhesus factor. See also Passive immunity.
Immunoglobulin	One of a group of proteins found in the blood which is able to react to foreign

matter or antigens as an antibody would.

Immunosuppression Suppression or inhibition of normal immune system responses. This may be a normal aspect of pregnancy, although in general use the term also applies where the immune system is suppressed with drugs, such as in transplant medicine.

Intercession By comparison with intervention this term, which is used by some holistic midwives, describes a natural or physiological substance, a lifestyle change or other action that is taken to prevent a problem or the need for medical intervention. This issue is discussed further in Chapter 9.

Intervention Any drug, procedure, test or other medical procedure used during any stage of childbirth. A routine intervention is one that is offered to all women (or all women in a particular group).

Intrapartum Describes the period of childbearing where the woman experiences labour and birth. This time is in turn divided into stages; the first stage describes the period whereby the woman experiences contractions as the cervix opens; the second stage describes the time from full opening of the cervix until the baby is born, and the third stage describes the birth of the placenta and the membranes.

Isoimmunization The process by which antibodies are produced in the body following detection of a foreign substance, in this case, the rhesus D antigen. NB: The terms 'isoimmunized' and 'sensitized' are used interchangeably.

Kleihauer test A test performed in a laboratory to attempt to determine whether fetal cells have entered the maternal circulation via fetomaternal haemorrhage. The technician adds a sample of the woman's blood to a dye that stains fetal haemoglobin and looks at this under a microscope to determine whether fetomaternal haemorrhage has occurred and to estimate the volume of this.

Medicalization   Describes the historical process whereby birth has become the remit of the medical profession, rather than primarily that of women and midwives. The important features of this process include: the movement of birth from home to hospital; the introduction of routine interventions into pregnancy and birth; and changes in authoritative knowledge concerning childbirth.

Optimal   Best, or ideal. In medical terms, used to describe the situation that is the best in terms of outcome or potential outcome.

Panacea   A universal remedy; a medicine for all diseases.

Paradigm   A set of ideas and beliefs which form a pattern; different paradigms describe different ways of approaching issues, which may ultimately lead to a variety of approaches and answers to the same question.

Paradox   A situation which seems absurd, even when it is generally accepted; something which conflicts with what is otherwise known about a situation.

Passive immunity   This is a form of immunity that may be given in one of two ways: (a) Babies have passive immunity via maternal antibodies which are passed through the placenta and breast milk; (b) Passive immunity may also be given where a person is injected with immunoglobulin from another person or, more rarely, an animal.

Pathological   Pertaining to disease, or the study of disease.

Philosophy	Relating to the love or study of knowledge. A person's philosophy describes their personal beliefs, values, understanding of and attitudes towards the world. Groups of people may have a shared philosophy in a particular area.
Physiological	Pertaining to the body; the study of the function of living things. This term is important in two respects here: (a) As opposed to pathological; (b) Describing the body's natural capacity to undertake the processes (e.g. birth) for which it was designed.
Postnatal	The period of the childbearing cycle that follows the baby's birth. Generally considered to last for several weeks or months.
Postpartum	See Postnatal.
Prophylaxis	Actions taken to prevent the occurrence of a disease or condition.
Qualitative	A form of research that generates theory (see Chapter 5).
Quantitative	A form of research grounded in scientific theory that tests ideas or propositions (see Chapter 5).
Rhesus disease	See Rhesus haemolytic disease of the newborn.
Rhesus factor	An antigen which is found in the blood of some people. The presence or absence of the rhesus factor will determine whether a person is rhesus positive or rhesus negative. So-called because it was originally identified in the rhesus monkey.
Rhesus haemolytic disease of the newborn	A disease caused in rhesus-positive newborn babies where a proportion of the baby's red blood cells are destroyed by a rhesus-negative mother's antibodies to the rhesus factor. The disease may be mild, moderate or severe.
Rhogam	This term is used by American midwives and midwives from some other countries

	as a generic term to describe anti-D immunoglobulin. It originates from a pharmaceutical form of anti-D with the same name.
Sensibilization	The state that exists in the body where antibodies are not detected by blood tests but exposure to rhesus-positive blood has occurred. A secondary immune response may be mounted in a subsequent pregnancy with a rhesus-positive baby. Although discussed in the medical literature, research into this concept is lacking.
Sensitization	See Isoimmunization.
Sub-optimal	Describes a situation where the outcomes are less than ideal; not the best possible (*cf.* Optimal).
Third stage (of labour)	See Intrapartum.
Transplacental haemorrhage	See Fetomaternal transfusion.
Vasodilatation	Widening (dilatation) of the blood vessels.

Bibliography

Alford, A. F. (1998). *The Phoenix Solution. Secrets of a Lost Civilization.* Hodder and Stoughton.

American College of Obstetricians and Gynecologists (1999). Prevention of Rh D alloimmunization: clinical management guidelines for obstetricians and gynecologists. *Int. J. Gynecol. Obstet.*, 66(1), 63–70.

Armstrong Fisher, S. S., Greiss, M. A. and Urbaniak, S. J. (1998). Prenatal determination of fetal RhD type by PCR-SSP using amniocyte DNA. Proceedings of the Consensus Conference on Anti-D Prophylaxis. *Br. J. Obstet. Gynaecol.*, 105(18), 24.

Ascari, W. Q., Allen, A. E., Baker, W. J. and Pollack, W. (1968). Rho(D) immune globulin (human) evaluation in women at risk of Rh immunization. *J. Am. Med. Assoc.*, 205(1), 1–4.

Ascari, W. Q., Levine, P. and Pollack, W. (1969). Incidence of maternal Rh immunization by ABO compatible and incompatible pregnancies. *Br. Med. J.*, 1, 399–401.

Bates, C. (1995). Can midwifery be both art and science? *Br. J. Midwifery*, 3(2), 67–8.

Baxter Healthcare Limited (1999). *Imported Supplies of Anti-D Safeguard Mothers-to-be.* Baxter Healthcare Limited.

Begley, C. M. (1998). Explaining postpartum haemorrhage; the value of a physiological third stage. In: *Returning Birth to Women. Challenging Policies and Practices* (P. Kennedy and J. Murphy-Lawless, eds). Centre for Women's Studies and Women's Education, Research and Resource Centre, University College Dublin.

Belenkey, M. F., Clinchy, B. M., Goldberger, N. R. and Tarule, J. M. (1997). *Women's Ways of Knowing; the Development of Self, Voice and Mind.* Basic Books.

Bennebrock Gravenhorst, J. (1989). Rhesus isoimmunisation. In: *Effective Care in Pregnancy and Childbirth* (I. Chalmers, M. Enkin and J. N. C. Keirse, eds), pp. 565–77. Oxford University Press.

BioProducts Laboratory (1996). *Anti-D* (Leaflet). BPL Elstree.

Bishop, G. J. and Krieger, V. I. (1969). One millilitre injections of Rho(D) immune globulin in prevention of Rh immunization. A further report on the clinical trial. *Med. J. Aust.*, 2, 171–4.

Blajchman, M. A., Maudsley, R. F., Uchida, I. *et al.* (1974).

Diagnostic amniocentesis and fetomaternal bleeding. *Lancet*, i, 993–4.

Bowman, J. M. and Pollock, J. M. (1978). Rh isoimmunisation during pregnancy: antenatal prophylaxis. *Can. Med. Assoc. J.*, **118**, 623–7.

Bryar, R. (1988). Midwifery and models of care. *Midwifery*, **4**, 111–17.

Chown, B., Duff, A. M., James, J. *et al.* (1969). Prevention of primary Rh immunization: First report of the Western Canadian Trial, 1966–1968. *Can. Med. Assoc. J.*, **100**, 1021–4.

Clarke, C. and Hussey, R. M. (1994). Decline in deaths from rhesus haemolytic disease of the newborn. *J. R. Coll. Phys. Lond.*, **28**, 310–11.

Clarke, C. A., Donahoe, W. T. A. and McConnell, R. B. (1963). Further experimental studies on the prevention of Rh haemolytic disease. *Br. Med. J.*, **1**, 979–84.

Clarke, C. A., Donohoe, W. T. A., Finn, R. *et al.* (Medical Research Council Working Party) (1971). Prevention of Rh haemolytic disease: final results of the 'high risk' clinical trial. *Br. Med. J.*, **217(2)**, 607–9.

Clarke, C. A., Finn, R., McConnell, R. B. and Sheppard, P. M. (1958). The protection offered by ABO incompatibility against erythroblastosis due to rhesus anti-D. *Int. Arch. Allergy*, **13**, 380.

Colquhoun, J. and Mann, R. (1986). The Hastings fluoridation experiment: science or swindle? *The Ecologist*, **16(6)**, 243–8.

Coombes, R. (1999). Midwives cautioned over risks of using untested blood product. *Nursing Times*, **95(24)**, 7.

Cooney, D. O. (1980). *Activated Charcoal*. Marcel Dekker, Inc.

Crowther, C. A. and Keirse, M. J. N. C. (1999). Anti-D administration in pregnancy for preventing rhesus alloimmunization. The Cochrane Library, Issue 4, Oxford, Update Software 1999.

Crowther, C. and Middleton, P. (1997). Anti-Rh-D prophylaxis postpartum. In: *Pregnancy and Childbirth Module of the Cochrane Database of Systematic Reviews* (J. P. Neilson, C. A. Crowther, E. D. Hodnett and G. Hofmeyr, eds). The Cochrane Collection, Issue 4, Oxford, Update Software 1997.

Cumberledge Report/Department of Health Expert Maternity Group (1992). *Maternity Services; Government Response to the Second Report from the Health Committee*. HMSO.

David, H. (1975). Doppler ultrasound and fetal activity. *Br. Med. J.*, **1**, 62–4.

Davis-Floyd, R. (1992). *Birth as an American Rite of Passage*. University of California Press.

Davis-Floyd, R. and Davis, E. (1996). Intuition as authoritative knowledge in midwifery and home birth. *Med. Anthropol. Q.*, 10(2), 237–69.

Davis-Floyd, R. and St John, G. (1998). *From Doctor to Healer: The Transformative Journey*. Rutgers University Press.

de Crespigny, L. and Davison, G. (1995). Anti-D administration in early pregnancy – time for a new protocol. *Aust. NZ J. Obstet. Gynecol.*, 35, 385–7.

du Bois, A., Quaas, L., Lorbeer, H. *et al.* (1991). Fetomaternal transfusion in relation to mode of delivery. Comparison of data from the DFG multicenter study 'Rhesus negative' (1965–70) with data from the Freiburg University Gynecologic Clinic (1989) (in German). *Zentralbl. Gynakol.*, 113(17), 927–33.

Dudok de Wit, C., Borst-Eilers, E., Weerdt, C. H. M. and Kloosterman, G. J. (1968). Prevention of Rh immunization. A controlled trial with a comparatively low dose of anti-D immunoglobulin. *Br. Med. J.*, 211(4), 477–9.

Dumasia, A., Kulkarni, S. and Joshi, S. H. (1989). Women receiving anti-Rho(D) immunoglobulin containing HIV antibodies (correspondence). *Lancet*, ii(8660), 459.

Durandy, A., Fisher, A. and Griscelli, C. (1981). Dysfunctions of pokeweed mitogen-stimulated T and B lymphocyte responses induced by gamma globulin therapy. *J. Clin. Invest.*, 67, 867.

Eason, C. (1999). *The Mother Link*. Ulysses Press/Seastone Books.

Edmunds, J. (1998). Prolonged labor – past and present. *Midwifery Today*, 46, 13–14.

El Halta, V. (1998). Taking the fear out of third stage. *Midwifery Today*, 48, 18–22.

Forchuk, C. and Roberts, J. (1993). How to critique qualitative research articles. *Can. J. Nursing Res.*, 25(4), 47–56.

Frey, A. (1997). *Understanding Diagnostic Tests in the Childbearing Year*, 6th edn. Labrys Press.

Gaskin, I. M. (1977). *Spiritual Midwifery*. The Book Publishing Company.

Gaskin, I. M. (1989). Rethinking rhogam. *Birth Gazette*, 6(1), 32–3.

Ghosh, S. and Murphy, W. G. (1994). Implementation of the rhesus prevention programme: a prospective study. *Scot. Med. J.*, 39(5), 147–9.

Gilling-Smith, C., Toozs-Hobson, P., Potts, D. J. *et al.* (1998). Failure to comply with anti-D prophylaxis recommendations in accident and emergency departments. Proceedings of the Consensus Conference on Anti-D Prophylaxis. *Br. J. Obstet. Gynaecol.*, 105(18), 24.

Ginesi, L. (1998). Maybe Descartes got it wrong. *Midwifery Today*, 47, 26–29, 71.

Glaser, B. and Strauss, A. (1967). *The Discovery of Grounded Theory: Strategies for Qualitative Research.* Aldine.

Graham, H. and Oakley, A. (1991). Competing ideologies of reproduction; medical and maternal perspective on pregnancy. In: *Concepts of Health, Illness and Disease. A Comparative Perspective* (C. Currer and M. Stacey, eds), pp. 97–116. Berg.

Harmon, P. (1987). Rhogam at 28 weeks. *Midwifery Today*, 4, 24–5.

Herb Research Foundation (1997). Herb Information Greenpaper: Zinc. Website: http://www.herbs.org/greenpapers/zinc.html

Herman, M., Kjellman, H. and Ljungggren, C. (1984). Antenatal prophylaxis of Rh isoimmunisation with 250 mg anti-D immunoglobulin. *Acta Obstet. Gynecol. Scand.*, 124, 1–15.

Hill Bailey, P. (1997). Finding your way around qualitative methods in nursing research. *J. Adv. Nursing*, 25, 18–22.

Hirzy, J. (1999). *Why Environmental Protection Agency's Headquarters Union of Scientists opposes Fluoridation.* National Treasury Employee's Union.

Hoffbrand, A. V., Lewis, S. M. and Tuddenham, E. G. D. (1999). *Postgraduate Haematology*, 4th edn. Butterworth Heinemann.

Holford, P. (1997). *The Optimum Nutrition Bible.* Piatkus.

Horey, D. (1995). Guidelines for the use of anti-D. *MA News*, 14, 17.

Howard, H. L., Martlew, V. J., McFadyn, I. R. and Clarke, C. A. (1997a). Preventing rhesus D haemolytic disease of the newborn by giving anti-D immunoglobulin: are the guidelines being adequately followed? *Br. J. Obstet. Gynaecol.*, 194, 37–41.

Howard, H. L., Martlew, V. J., McFadyn, I. R. *et al.* (1997b). Current use of anti-D immunoglobulin in preventing rhesus hemolytic disease. *Contemporary Rev. Obstet. Gynecol.*, 9(3), 181–8.

Huchet, J., Dallemagne, S., Huchet, C. *et al.* (1987). The antepartum use of anti-D immunoglobulin in rhesus negative women. Parallel evaluation of fetal blood cells passing through the placenta. The results of a multicentre trial carried out in the region of Paris. *J. Gynecol. Obstet. Biol. Reprod. (Paris)*, **16**, 101–11.

Huggon, A. M. and Watson, D. P. (1993). Use of anti-D in an accident and emergency department. *Arch. Emergency Med.*, **10(4)**, 306–9.

Hughes, R. G., Craig, J. L., Murphy, W. G. *et al.* (1994). Causes and clinical consequences of rhesus (D) haemolytic disease of the newborn: a study of a Scottish population, 1985–1990. *Br. J. Obstet. Gynaecol.*, **101(4)**, 297–300.

Hughes-Jones, N. C., Ellis, M., Ivona, J. *et al.* (1971). Anti-D concentrations in mother and child in haemolytic disease of the newborn. *Vox Sang.*, **124**, 135.

Huntley, A. (1999). Midwives in cyberspace. *Midwifery Today*, **49**, 20–21.

Inch, S. (1982). *Birthrights. A Parents' Guide to Modern Childbirth.* Hutchinson.

Jacobs, W. (1956). The use of bioflavinoid compounds in the prevention or reduction in severity of erythroblastosis fetalis. *Surg. Obstet. Gynecol.*, **August,** 233–6.

Jacobs, W. (1960). Further experience with bioflavinoid compounds in Rh immunized women. *Surg. Obstet. Gynecol.*, **January,** 33–4.

Jacobs, W. (1965). Citrus bioflavinoid compounds in Rh-immunized gravidas: results of a ten year study. *Am. J. Obstet. Gynecol.*, **25(5)**, 648–9.

Jowitt, M. (1993). *Childbirth Unmasked.* Self-Publishing Association.

Katz, J. (1969). Transplacental passage of fetal red cells in abortion; increased incidence after curettage and effect of oxytocic drugs. *Br. Med. J.*, **214(4)**, 84–6.

Kirchebner, C., Solder, E. and Schonitzer, D. (1994). Prevention of rhesus incompatibility and viral safety (in German). *Infusionsther. Transfusionmed.*, **24(4)**, 281.

Kitzinger, S. (1988). *Freedom and Choice in Childbirth.* Penguin.

Lachman, E., Hingley, S. M., Bates, G. *et al.* (1977). Detection and measurement of fetomaternal haemorrhage; serum alpha-protein and Kleihauer technique. *Br. Med. J.*, **240(1)**, 1377–9.

Lambley, J. (1985). Ultrasound debate. *New Generation*, **4**, 5–6.

Lark, S. M. (1999). *The Woman's Health Companion.* Celestial Arts. **NB:** Sections from the 'Foods to eat for good health' chapter, which is referred to in Chapter 9, are available online: http://www.healthy.net/library/books/lark/fdstoeat.htm

Lawrence Beech, B. A. and Robinson, J. (1996). *Ultrasound? Unsound.* AIMS.

Lee, D. and Rawlinson, V. I. (1995). Multicentre trial of antepartum low-dose anti-D immunoglobulin. *Trans. Med.*, **5**, 15–19.

Levine, P., Katzin, E. M. and Burnham, L. (1941). Isoimmunisation in pregnancy. Its possible bearing on the etiology of erythroblastosis fetalis. *J. Am. Med. Assoc.*, **116**, 825–7.

Magee, B. (1988). *The Great Philosophers.* OUP.

Maisels, M. J. (1992). Advice not to clamp cord immediately. *Obstet. Gynecol. News*, **19(24)**, 4.

Malviya, A. N., Tripathy, S., Chaudhary, K. *et al.* (1989). The anti-D vaccine episode; lessons for everyone in the HIV field. *CARC Calling*, **2**, 12.

Mayne, S., Parker, J. H., Dodds, S. D. *et al.* (1997). Rate of RhD sensitisation before and after implementation of a community based antenatal prophylaxis programme. *Br. Med. J.*, **315**, 1588.

McSweeney, E., Kirkham, J., Vinall, P. *et al.* (1998). An audit of anti-D sensitisation in Yorkshire. *Br. J. Obstet. Gynaecol.*, **105**, 1091–4.

Medical Research Council (1974). Report of a Working Party on the use of anti-D immunoglobulin for the prevention of isoimmunization of Rh-negative women during pregnancy. Controlled trial of various dosages in suppression of Rh sensitization following pregnancy. *Br. Med. J.*, **2**, 72–80.

Meisel, H., Reip, A. and Faltus, B. (1995). Transmission of hepatitis C virus to children and husbands by women infected with contaminated anti-D immunoglobulin. *Lancet*, **345(8589)**, 1209–11.

Midwives' Alliance of North America (MANA) (1998). *Statement of Values and Ethics.* MANA.

Miller, D., Hamlington, J., Cunningham, J. *et al.* (1998). Prenatal detection of rhesus D by maternal blood sampling and RT-PCR amplification of D-specific messenger RNA. Proceedings of the Consensus Conference on Anti-D Prophylaxis. *Br. J. Obstet. Gynaecol.*, **105(18)**, 24.

Mollison, P. L., Barron, S. L., Bowley, C. C. *et al.* (1974). Controlled trial of various anti-D dosages in suppression of Rh sensitisation following pregnancy: report to the Medical Research Council by the Working Party on the use of anti-D immunoglobulin for the prevention of isoimmunization of Rh-negative women during pregnancy. *Br. Med. J.*, **2**, 75–80.

Morley, G. M. (1998). Cord closure; can hasty clamping injure the newborn? *Obstet. Gynecol. Management*, July, 29–30, 33–34, 36. Available online: www.gentlebirth.org/archives/hastyclamping.html

Morse, J. M. (1992). *Qualitative Health Research*. Sage Publications.

Nevanlinner, H. R. and Vainio, T. (1956). The influence of mother–child ABO incompatibility on Rh immunisation. *Vox Sang.*, **1**, 26.

Norager Stern, P. (1985). Using grounded theory methods in nursing research. In: *Qualitative Research Methods in Nursing* (M. M. Leininger, ed.), pp. 65–81. Grune and Stratton.

Odent, M. (1996). Land food... sea food... brain food. *Midwifery Today*, **40**, 18–20.

Odent, M. (1998). Don't manage the third stage of labour! *Practising Midwife*, **1**(9), 31–3.

Odent, M. (1999). Untitled commentary. *MIDIRS Midwifery Digest*, **9**(4), 525.

Olovnikova, N. L., Belkina, E. V., Drize, N. I. *et al.* (1997). Immunoglobulin G monoclonal human anti-rhesus Rho(D) to prevent rhesus incompatibility (in Russian). *Klin. Med. (Mosk.)*, **75**(7), 39–43.

Page, L. (1997). Evidence-based practice in midwifery: a virtual revolution? *J. Clin. Effect.*, **2**(1), 10–13.

Pollack, W., Gorman, J. G., Hagel, H. J. *et al.* (1968). Antibody mediated immune suppression to the Rh factor: animal models suggesting mechanism of action. *Transfusion*, **8**, 134.

Prendeville, W. J., Harding, J., Elbourne, D. R. *et al.* (1988). The Bristol third stage trial; active versus physiological management of third stage of labour. *Br. Med. J.*, **297**, 1295–1300.

Reilly, M. and Lawlor, E. (1999). A likelihood-based method of identifying contaminated lots of blood product. *Int. J. Epidemiol.*, **28**(4), 787–92.

Robbins, J. (1987). *Diet for a New America: How Your Food Choices Affect Your Health, Happiness and the Future of Life on Earth*. Stillpoint.

Robbins, J. (1996). *Reclaiming Our Health*. H. J. Kramer.

Robertson, A. (1997). The pain of labor. *Midwifery Today*, **39**, 19–21, 40–42.

Robertson, J. G. and Holmes, C. M. (1969). A clinical trial of anti-Rho(D) immunoglobulin in the prevention of Rho(D) immunization. *J. Obstet. Gynaecol. Br. Commonwealth*, **76**, 252–9

Robson, S. C., Lee, D. and Urbaniak, S. (1998). Anti-D immunoglobulin in RhD prophylaxis. *Br. J. Obstet. Gynaecol.,* **105,** 129–34.

Rogers, J., Wood, J., McCandlish, R. *et al.* (1998). Active versus expectant management of third stage of labour; the Hinchingbrooke randomised controlled trial. *Lancet,* **351,** 693–9.

Romm, A. V. (1999). Rho(D) immune globulin: pros, cons, indications and alternatives. *Birth Gazette,* **15(2),** 18–21.

Royal College of Midwives (1999). Anti-D update. *RCM Midwives Journal,* November 1999 mid-month supplement.

Safe, S. H. and Gaido, K. (1998). Phytoestrogens and anthropogenic estrogen compounds. *Environ. Toxicol. Chem.,* **17(1)** , 119–26.

Saha, A. (1998). Women should be counselled about source of anti-D immunoglobulin (letter). *Br. Med. J.,* **316,** 1164.

Schlensker, K. H. and Kruger, A. A. (1996). Results of postpartum prophylaxis 1967–1990 (in German). *Geburtshilfe Frauenheilkd,* **56(9),** 494–500.

Shelton, H. M. (1995). *The Myth of Medicine.* Cool Hand Communications.

Siddiqui, J. (1994). A philosophical exploration of midwifery knowledge. *Br. J. Midwifery,* **2(9),** 419–22.

Standing Medical Advisory Committee (1976). *Haemolytic Disease of the Newborn.* Department of Health and Social Security.

Standing Medical Advisory Committee (1976 – addendum 1981). *Memorandum on Haemolytic Disease of the Newborn.* Department of Health and Social Security.

Stenchever, M. A., Davies, I. J., Weisman, R. and Gross, S. (1970). Rho(D) immunoglobulin: a double blind clinical trial. *Am. J. Obstet. Gynecol.,* **106(2),** 316–17.

Stewart, M. (1999). Untitled commentary. *MIDIRS Midwifery Digest,* **9(4),** 525.

Stine, L. E., Phelan, J. P., Do, R. W. *et al.* (1985). Update on external version performed at term. *Obstet. Gynecol.,* **65,** 642–6.

Sutton, J. (2000). Birth without active pushing and a physiological second stage of labour. *Practising Midwife,* **3(4),** 32–4.

Thrash, A. M. and Thrash, C. L. (1981). *Nutrition for Vegetarians.* New Lifestyle Books.

Thrash, A. M. and Thrash, C. L. (1988). *Charcoal.* New Lifestyle Books.

Tovey, L. A. D. (1986). Haemolytic disease of the newborn – the changing scene. *Brit. J. Obst. Gynaecol.,* **93(9),** 960–66.

Tovey, L. A. D., Townley, A., Stevenson, B. *et al.* (1983). The Yorkshire antenatal anti-D immunoglobulin trial in primigravidae. *Lancet*, ii, 244–6.

Urbaniak, S. (1998). Proceedings of the Consensus Conference on Anti-D prophylaxis. *Br. J. Obstet. Gynaecol.*, 105(18), 24.

van Dijk, B. (1997). Preventing RhD haemolytic disease of the newborn (editorial). *Br. Med. J.*, 315, 1480–81.

Vos, G. H. (1967). The effect of external version on antenatal immunization by the Rh factor. *Vox Sang.*, 12, 390–96.

Walshe, K. (1995). Given in evidence. *Health Service J.*, 29 June, 14–15.

White, C. A., Visscher, R. D., Visscher, H. C. and Wade, M. D. (1970). Rho(D) immune prophylaxis: a double blind co-operative study. *Obstet. Gynecol.*, 36(3), 341–6.

Whitfield, C. R., Raafat, A. and Urbaniak, S. J. (1997). Underreporting of mortality from RhD haemolytic disease in Scotland and its implications: retrospective review. *Br. Med. J.*, 315, 1504–5.

Wickham, S. (1998). Rhogam: do midwives hold the evidence? *Midwifery Today*, 46, 34–5.

Wickham, S. (1999a). Anti-D: an informed choice? Part 1. *Practising Midwife*, 2(5), 18–19.

Wickham, S. (1999b). Anti-D: an informed choice? Part 2. *Practising Midwife*, 2(6), 38–9.

Wickham, S. (1999c). Further thoughts on the third stage. *Practising Midwife*, 2(10), 14–15. (Reprinted in *MIDIRS Midwifery Digest*, 10(2), 204–5.)

Wickham, S. (1999d). Evidence-informed mMidwifery 1: what is evidence-informed midwifery? *Midwifery Today*, 51, 42–3.

Woodrow, J. C. and Donahoe, W. T. A. (1968). Rh-immunization by pregnancy; results of a survey and their relevance to prophylactic therapy. *Br. Med. J.*, 4, 139–44.

Woodrow, J. C., Clarke, C. A., McConnell, R. B. *et al.* (1971). Prevention of Rh-haemolytical disease: results of the Liverpool 'low-risk' clinical trial. *Br. Med. J.*, 2, 610–12.

Yap, P. L. (1997). Viral transmission by blood products: a perspective of events covered by the recent tribunal of enquiry into the Irish Blood Transfusion Board. *Irish Med. J.*, 90(3), 84, 86, 88.

Zipursky, A. and Israels, L. G. (1967). The pathogenesis and prevention of Rh immunization. *Can. Med. Assoc. J.*, 97(21), 1245–57.

Index

9 780750 652322

Lightning Source UK Ltd.
Milton Keynes UK
UKHW020630091121
393664UK00013B/886